May your - full of fresh & chocolate. Love, Lindsay M. Reinholt 4/26/16

Meant to Eat:
A Practical Guide to Developing a Healthy Relationship with Food

LINDSAY M. REINHOLT

Copyright © 2016 Lindsay Reinholt

All rights reserved. No part of this book may be reproduced in any form or
by any electronic or mechanical means, including information storage and
retrieval systems, without permission in writing from the author. For more
information, contact Lindsay Reinholt at lindsay@lindsayreinholt.com.

The content of this book is for general instruction only. Each person's
physical, emotional, and spiritual condition is unique. The instruction in this
book is not intended to replace or interrupt the reader's relationship with a
physician or other professional. Please consult your doctor for matters
pertaining to your specific health and diet.

ISBN-10: 0692675825
ISBN-13: 978-0692675823

DEDICATION

This book is dedicated to Mitch, Winnie, and the beautiful baby in my belly.
I love you with all of my heart.

CONTENTS

ACKNOWLEDGMENTS

I want to thank the various people that helped make this dream of mine a reality. First, I would have never written this book without the loving support of my wonderful husband Mitch, who believed in me even when I was unsure. Next, I'd like to thank my editor, Christine Cummings, for using her scrutinizing eye to perfect my writing without changing my message or voice. I would also like to thank my friend and photographer, Lena Winn, for the time and energy she put into getting the perfect headshot while minimizing my growing pregnant belly. In addition, I must thank my health coaching clients, who teach me just as much as I teach them. And lastly, I am so indebted to the various friends and family members who supported me in this journey, by doing everything from reading and giving feedback to offering kind words of encouragement when I felt overwhelmed. I appreciate all of you so much. Thank you.

PART ONE:
STOP DIETING, START LIVING

1. INTRODUCTION

There is no sincerer love than the love for food.

--George Bernard Shaw

I am in love with food. I love how it looks. I love how it smells. And, of course, I love how it tastes. Food is fun, inspiring, and sensual. It connects me to my roots and compels me to be a better person. If it is cold outside, food makes me warm; if it is hot, food can cool me off. It gives me a creative outlet and helps me to take care of the people around me. Eating is one of the few things that I must do every day that I thoroughly enjoy every time I do it. The culinary world provides unlimited possibilities—I never have to be bored. I truly *love* food.

I have not always felt this way. For many years, I felt at odds with my love of food, fighting guilt and confusion over how and what I chose to eat. It seemed to me that enjoying delicious food could not coexist with living a healthy lifestyle, so I was in a never-ending conflict of which side to choose.

I was at war with my body. I talked down to it, starved it, stuffed it, shamed it, and truly abused it. Like many young people, girls in particular, I learned at a young age that my body was not good enough, and that it had to be my fault. I set off on years of attempts to remedy my "problem." I tried everything from counting calories to over-exercising. I even forced myself to get sick a handful of times, all in an attempt to achieve a more ideal body and fix my inability to control myself with food. I was never diagnosed with a full-blown eating disorder, but I knew enough to know that I was on a bad path. Something needed to change.

My preoccupation with weight continued until two marvelous things happened that changed everything for me: (1) I enrolled in the Institute for Integrative Nutrition®, where I studied to become a health coach and (2) I became pregnant with my first child. These two events, which actually happened concurrently, drastically changed my relationship with food. I began viewing food as my friend, not the enemy, and my body as something to cherish and nurture, not to hate. Even as my belly was growing and the number on the scale was increasing, I found that I was so taken with the beautiful miracle of pregnancy that the weight didn't concern me. My body wasn't just mine anymore, and its purpose was no longer to look a certain way. In fact, it was now here to provide a healthy home to my growing baby. I knew, in order to do that, I needed to make some drastic changes to my relationship with food. I also knew that if I continued to put the health of the baby and me first, my eating would reflect that both before and after the birth, and postpartum weight loss wouldn't need to be a concern.

My Problem is the Problem of Many People, Maybe Even You

Unfortunately, I am not alone in this struggle. Many people deal with issues that come from an unhealthy relationship with food. We have an abundance of food options and information, but we are more confused than ever. Every other day, there are new stories in the media about the latest and greatest diet that is going to help you drop the pounds fast, yet many people don't even know how to recognize when they are hungry and full. Cycling between dieting and deprivation and then overindulgence and guilt steals the enjoyment that people are meant to have during the eating experience.

And maybe the biggest problem of all is that this way of eating offers no respite. The moment we finish one diet, we are often already thinking ahead to when we will inevitably have to start the next. Studies show that when people end their diets, they often gain more weight than they lost in the first place. Dieting really does more harm than good.

Fluctuating between overindulgence and deprivation not only adds weight but can have negative psychological impacts, as well. You start to view food as the enemy, and every diet is a new battle plan. This mentality also damages your self-esteem and makes body-acceptance almost impossible.

What if Things Could Change For You?

This book will forever change your relationship with food and your body. You will learn how to quit dieting and banish deprivation, guilt, and self-hate forever. In addition, you will likely experience effortless weight loss and maintenance, body acceptance, and a whole new level of self-love and compassion. Furthermore, you will learn to enjoy a variety of new foods in a more satisfying and pleasurable way than ever before.

I know because I did it, and you can too. You can turn away from the lies you've been told by the media, your friends, family, and society. You can learn to embrace a way of eating that is natural, flexible, and healthy. As a result, you can feel and look your best.

I wrote this book to help you do just that. There are all kinds of diet books out there preaching that their way of eating is the best, but not enough of them are promoting a healthy, natural, and mindful way of eating. What you will read in the coming pages is not glamorous. You won't lose fifteen pounds in fifteen days, but what you will learn will transform your life. When I share this message with people, they almost universally say the same thing, "That makes so much sense!"

What You Can Expect

This book will walk you through the process of turning away from your old ways and embracing a healthy, sustainable relationship with food. It is a lifestyle change, and that change needs to start in your mind. In Part One, I will present my argument for why diets not only don't work, but are harmful to a person's health. After that, we will take a look at how we were actually meant to eat—mindfully eating real food that feeds both the body and soul in a way that is flexible and enjoyable. The next two parts constitute the "how-to" part of the book. Lasting change has to start from within, so that is how it is set up here. In Part Two, I will lead you through the step-by-step process of how to break from the diet mentality and embrace a healthy relationship with food from a *psychological* perspective. Part Three is all about implementation.

I hope you are looking forward to this process. Remember, this journey is *yours*—not mine, not your spouse's, and not your friends'. Be willing to take your time, feel vulnerable, and be open to change. If you do this, your world will be rocked in a very awesome way. It's time to learn how you were always *meant to eat*. Let's get started.

2. THE MYTH OF DIETING: YOU'VE BEEN FED A LIE

How many times have you been at an event when someone has revealed that they are on a new diet? Maybe they began raving about how easy it was, how great they felt, and the pounds that they were losing. Or maybe they began complaining about how terrible they felt—starved, tired, and frustrated. Maybe you've even been that person before. I know that I have.

There is a mystical allure of dieting. There's always a glimmer of hope as you set out on a new program. *Maybe this time will be the time that I get the body I've always dreamed of!* There's something exciting about having a set of shiny new rules to follow, something comforting about parameters. Usually we get caught up in the promise of a new diet. Maybe you know someone who experienced success, you saw the author of the diet on the news, or you read a testimonial online.

Unfortunately, this hype is usually short-lived. While dieting, people usually under-eat and become overly hungry, cranky, and bored with their food choices. Frequently, the pounds don't come off as quickly as the dieter had hoped. We all know that feeling of standing on the scale as the machine takes a moment to evaluate our weight. In those few seconds, I know that I've said a prayer or two hoping to see a certain dream number and definitely nothing higher than my last weigh-in. How many times have you done the same, only to be disappointed when the number glaring back at you has screamed, "You didn't do good enough!"?

At different times in my life before discovering true health, I would get into the habit of weighing myself multiple times in the day, hoping that my weight would dip magically at different hours. Sometimes, I would see a pound or two difference, but that was almost always a reflection of water weight, a meal I just ate, or whether I had used the bathroom yet that day. I put so much stock in what some stupid piece of machinery said about my worth!

Even when I was successful at losing weight, I always put it back on—sometimes quickly and sometimes over the course of several months, but it always crept back. And I am not alone in this. Traci Mann, expert on the psychology of eating and author of the book *Secrets from the Eating Lab*, did a review of studies that looked at how effective diets are in the long-term. What she found was that on average, after a few years, diet participants were only able to keep off two pounds of the weight they lost. If that seems depressing, consider that around forty-percent of the people studied actually weighed *more* at their follow-ups than they did before embarking on the diet in the first place. In each of these studies, there was a control group which didn't diet at all. These people only gained one pound over the same period of time. All of that effort and the difference was only three pounds between the dieters and non-dieters, and many of the dieters were worse off than their non-dieting counterparts![1]

Think about it—the "promise" of a new diet is really quite empty. We live at a time when anyone can prove virtually anything by just getting the right researcher to run the study, skew the results, find the right participant, and catch them before they put the weight back on. And the truth is, diet companies don't want their products to help you lose weight and keep it off for good. They are built on the premise that you will fail *eventually*; that way, they have a steady stream of repeat customers.

One of the worst things about dieting is that it breeds a whole host of negative behaviors and thought patterns. Society glorifies the skinny shape, and food choices are often considered synonymous with a person's strength of character. People assume that if a person is overweight, the blame falls squarely on their shoulders. *That person is gluttonous and has no self-control,* many think. I will get into this later when I discuss body image, but it's a sad truth that discrimination based on weight is still considered socially acceptable in many circles. Fat shaming happens all around us, in all kinds of settings, by people who would never make a negative comment about someone's gender, race, or religion. Yet we find it perfectly okay to both privately and publicly ridicule people based on their body size. In fact, being overweight may affect your ability to get into grad school[2] or be hired for a job.[3]

We internalize these messages that are constantly bombarding us and assume that we must be bad people if we are unable to control our eating choices. And so we become guilty, and that guilt makes us feel even worse about ourselves. When we beat ourselves up with constant negative self-talk, we are less likely to treat our bodies in a way that is body loving and honoring. *What's the point of eating healthfully if I don't love my body anyways?* And so it continues. It's truly a horrible cycle.

Maybe you've wondered if you could be successful if you just had a bit more willpower. Unfortunately, it is not as simple as that. As Traci Mann suggests, using willpower with food is different from using willpower in other areas of our lives.

For example, willpower can be effective when it comes time to doing certain things that you'd rather not do but that you will yourself to do nonetheless. An example of this would be if you were in school and you were presented with the option to study for an upcoming exam or go out with your friends. Going out is certainly more fun that studying, but the knowledge of how you would fare on your exam without studying is a motivating force to get you to stay home and study instead. Once your friends take off, your decision is made. No more willpower needed. It takes only one instance of strong willpower to succeed here.

Food, on the other hand, is a different matter entirely. Imagine you are at home on a Sunday afternoon and you have a bag of chips in the pantry that is calling your name. You first resist, knowing that you are not hungry and shouldn't eat the chips. Yay for you! Suddenly, though, all you can think about are those darn chips. You perform another monumental act of willpower and get a glass of water, hoping to distract yourself and pop down in front of the TV. Good job again! But sitting in your favorite chair and watching TV makes you think about eating because you often eat while watching TV. So you start thinking about those chips again.

This could go on and on, until you cannot take it any more and you succumb to the chips. You probably will then beat yourself up about not having enough willpower and giving in. *I am so weak!*, you may think. But the reality is that you are quite strong. You resisted valiantly several times, but unfortunately the deck was stacked against you.[1]

Self-control around food is unique and different from self-control in other areas of our lives. When you add dieting (restriction of food) to the mix, it makes it even more challenging. When you set out on a diet, your stress levels increase for a variety of reasons, some of them due to how you are eating (not enough), and some of them due to the psychological aspects of dieting.

The problem is, when it comes to willpower, stress is not your friend. Stress has a negative effect on the functioning of the prefrontal cortex, the part of the brain responsible for higher-order thinking, reasoning, and decision-making.[4] So you are less capable, cognitively, of making good choices about what you are going to eat.

Another side effect of dieting is the fact that when food is restricted from the diet, it actually becomes even more appetizing than it was beforehand. I'm sure you can relate with this. When you are off-diet, junk food is no big deal, but the second you go on a diet, it suddenly looks, smells, and tastes *amazing*. Scientists have actually studied this phenomenon and found that when on a diet, our brains actually change, making food appear more desirable. On top of that, the reward centers in the brain become more responsive, making that brownie even more gratifying when you eat it.[5]

Not only are there neurological reasons why dieting doesn't work, but there are hormonal ones, too. Quite simply, our bodies are ridiculously smart. When we suddenly and drastically change our diets through restriction, our bodies sort of freak out and think that food suddenly is scarce. *I must be starving,* your body thinks. Hormones are then produced that make you feel hungrier, so you eat more. In addition, your metabolism is down-regulated so that you burn fewer calories. It's your body's way of sustaining itself. Your body has no way of knowing that you are surrounded by food options but are just *choosing* not to eat. It thinks that it has to do everything in its power to get you to seek and eat food, store that food as fat, and keep any body fat it already has from going away.

Beyond that, there is increasing evidence that dieting, especially doing several diets during one's life, can make it increasingly harder to lose weight in the future. In fact, studies show that dieting is a predictor of accelerated weight gain and becoming overweight.

Some people explain their weight struggles by saying that it's genetic. *My mom was big, so I will be big.* Yes, genetics can certainly predispose you to a larger frame, but dieting can also play a pivotal role.

In an interesting study, a researcher in Finland looked at over 2,000 sets of twins. One member of each set was a dieter and the other was not. Commonly held belief would tell us that the twin that watched their weight and dieted would be the thinner of the two, right? Wrong. The dieter was actually two to three times more likely than the other twin to be overweight, and the chances of weight gain increased with each diet they embarked on. The more they dieted, the more likely they were to become overweight.[6]

Your body doesn't want to die, so it keeps making adjustments to keep the weight on. Plus, if you are *repeatedly* making it think that you are starving, it will want to keep putting layers of fat on as insurance for the next inevitable "famine." Better safe than sorry in the world of survival.

In addition, sometimes dieting drives us to self-sabotage. We get tired of following the rules all the time, so we lash out and do what feels good—eat. I see this most often with my clients after they "mess up" a little, i.e. they give in and have a cookie from the break room. The rest of the day they figure that they blew their diet, so they eat whatever they want and tell themselves they will go back to eating healthfully tomorrow.

Sometimes this comes as a result of frustration with a lack of results. If you've been on a diet for two weeks and haven't lost any weight, you may figure, *What the heck? Saying "no" to all my favorite foods isn't helping me lose weight anyways! Bring on the doughnuts!* When all the focus is on restriction and weight loss as the ultimate goal, this kind of behavior is really quite understandable. And so we need a paradigm shift.

3. WHAT WE WERE MEANT TO EAT

In order to truly fix a problem, you must get to the root
of it, and the root of our food problem is that we have lost touch
with how we were meant to eat. There are many theories about
the specifics of what human beings are supposed to eat based on
all kinds of interesting research, but what most everyone agrees
on is that the Standard American Diet is *not* the answer. Based
on the evidence I presented in the previous chapter, I will go a
step further and suggest that the on-and-off dieting cycle is not
ideal for human well-being, either. *Well, that's all well and good,*
you may be thinking, *but how and what are we supposed to eat?* The
short answer? The way we were meant to eat. The longer
answer? Read on.

I believe that there are some general principles that make
up how humans were meant to eat—*what* foods we should be
eating, *when* those eating episodes should be taking place, and *how*
we should actually be doing the act of consuming food. In
addition, I believe there are some ways in which humans use
food today which are not how it is meant to be used.

First, let's specifically look at *what* we should be eating.
In a nutshell, we should be eating foods that nourish our minds,

bodies, and souls. Our food choices should make us feel good—emotionally, philosophically and physically.

Food Should Make Us Feel Good Emotionally

Our food choices should be ones that we feel good about. Food should make us happy! For me, sometimes that is a meal that is a rainbow of colors—lots of fruits and vegetables. Other times, it is something that brings back a feeling of comfort or love—my grandmother's caramel apple pie is a perfect example of this. In addition, the look on my daughter's face when I give her a banana wonderfully demonstrates happiness found in food. She totally lights up, smiling and kicking her legs like crazy and happily saying, "Nana!", right up to the moment she hungrily chomps down on the sweet fruit.

Unfortunately, for many people, experiences in their past have left negative emotional connections with food. Maybe the adults in their lives criticized their eating when they were little or forced them to eat foods that weren't palatable to them. It's also possible that their parents restricted their eating in an effort to control weight. Children often grow up watching their parents' own struggles with food, weight, and body image, and that can have devastating effects on how they learn to view themselves. Maybe they turned to food as an emotional outlet or escape during periods of stress or change. When enough of these instances happen in a person's life, the person begins to associate certain foods or eating events with the negative emotions of shame, stress, and worthlessness. Oftentimes, this manifests itself in many unhealthy ways regarding food.

The good news is that food was meant to be a pleasure in life. It doesn't have to be a source of stress, preoccupation, shame, and mistrust. When you follow your body's signals and eat the foods that both taste good and feel good in the body, your food will start making you feel better emotionally, as well.

Food Should Make Us Feel Good Philosophically

Our food choices should align with our beliefs. Traditions related to food are an important part of almost every religion. Certain meals are part of religious holidays, such as the Passover meal for the Jewish faith. Christians take Communion, a symbolic "meal" made up of bread and wine that is meant to represent Jesus's Last Supper. Some religions place restrictions on what foods are appropriate for consumption by followers and even what foods will connect you more with God.

Even our non-religious beliefs may affect our eating preferences. People that take a stand against animal cruelty or are concerned with the many aspects of how animals are raised from a health or environmental perspective may make the choice not to consume meat or other animal products. Supporting local farmers as opposed to large agricultural corporations motivates many to shop at farmers' markets, join CSAs, and grow their own food. "Locavore" is a term that has sprung up to describe this eating preference. Your beliefs about your own health and wellness may lead you to make certain eating decisions, too.

Food is an incredibly poignant way of expressing our beliefs in an outward manner. These choices and traditions bind us to others who share our beliefs and make us part of a community. Considering your faith and philosophies when making food choices is a healthy approach that makes this aspect of your life more aligned with the other aspects. Reflect on your beliefs about the world around you and whether or not the way you eat fits in with those beliefs. If it doesn't, then this may be something to change.

Food Should Make Us Feel Good Physically

Ah yes, you may be thinking, *this is where she is going to give me the "nutrition talk."* There is a reason I reserved this section for after I discussed the pleasures of eating and the effect our beliefs have on our eating choices. I think it is important to work on those first, but leaving out nutrition would be irresponsible of me. Yes, I advocate balance and eating what you want, even if it isn't always the most "healthy" from a nutritional perspective, but I would be remiss to say that nutrition doesn't matter. It does. It affects all of our bodily processes for the good or the bad. I sometimes say that every food either moves us closer to wellness or further from it. That's not to say that you have to abstain from all sugar, fat, processed food, etc. In fact, in some situations, eating something that many nutritionists would call "unhealthy" may actually be the *healthier* choice from an emotional or social perspective, even if it isn't the most nutritious option. If you love your mom's pumpkin pie and she loves making it for the family to enjoy together on Thanksgiving, you shouldn't feel like you are being unhealthy for eating a slice. In fact, eating it may be a healthy option when you do it in the context of a traditional family gathering, you thoroughly enjoy every bite, and you stop when you are full.

My point is that "health" means a lot of things to a lot of people, but most agree that what you choose to put into your body will have consequences, intended or unintended, good or bad. Many of us, especially those coming from a past of habitual dieting and restriction, have been beaten over the head by nutrition. *Eat this! Don't eat that! Not too much! Carbs are good! Carbs are bad! Fat is good! Fat is bad! Everyone should be vegetarian/gluten-free/paleo/low-carb!* And so on. Unfortunately, much of this information is confusing, contradictory, and, sometimes, flat-out wrong.

Bio-Individuality

First of all, I do not believe that one specific diet is the "right" diet for everyone. (By "diet" here, I mean "way of eating.") In my practice with clients, I teach them about bio-individuality, the concept that we are all different and our food choices should reflect that. We have different food preferences, genetics, family histories, and nutritional needs, and we live in different environments. What is nourishing to me may actually be unhealthy to you, and vice versa; and what is appropriate for me to eat at this moment in my life may not be the way I should eat five years from now.

This approach is flexible and intuitive. It means that your diet shifts along with the rest of your life when changes come. It also renders useless the habit of comparing yourself to others. How can you compare when what *you* need nutritionally is different from what those around you need? Following that logic, how can you feel guilty or upset with yourself when you choose foods that are different from those of your friends and family? If you've tried kale a million ways and have hated it every time, there's no need to feel like some sort of failure. Yes, kale is currently a superstar of the nutrition world, but it is not a cure-all for everyone's nutritional needs, and there are plenty of other good options out there for getting the same nutrients found in it.

We must be ready to change our eating styles and food choices if our bodies require it. Prior to getting pregnant, I was in the habit of eating a big serving of vegetables and some sort of meat at most of my dinners. It made me feel satisfied, strong, and energized, and it was easy for me to plan for and prepare. As I progressed through my first trimester of pregnancy, though, I began to notice a shift in my preferences. As is very common for pregnant women, I developed an aversion to several foods, including my tried-and-true meat and vegetable dinners. I found myself unable to eat much at dinner, feeling nauseated by the idea of these foods (especially raw meat and Brussels sprouts!), and pushing my plate away. And so, during my pregnancy, especially at the beginning, I ate much less of these foods and incorporated more starchy, carbohydrate-rich foods into my diet, and I didn't feel guilty about it at all. In the moments when those vegetables or meats sounded good, I ate them, and I continued taking my prenatal vitamins and eating other nutritionally rich foods to compensate. I made my diet work for me instead of forcing myself to eat foods my body was rejecting.

Whole Foods

So, which foods are most likely to make you feel good physically? In my opinion, and the opinion of many experts, the best approach is a whole-foods approach. Whole foods are those foods that are available in nature, not manufactured in a lab, and that are as close to their natural form as possible. They don't come in special packages with lengthy labels, and if they *do* have an ingredient list, that list reads like a recipe, not a science experiment. At the grocery store, these foods items tend to be housed around the perimeter of the store, while the processed, non-whole foods are stocked in the shelves in the middle. Fruits, vegetables, meat, fish, dairy, natural oils and fats, and whole grains all fall into the category of whole foods.

One of the most beautiful things about a whole-foods approach is that it is simple. There are no concerns with analyzing macro- and micro-nutrient levels (i.e. having a certain amount of protein versus carbs or looking too closely at the vitamins and minerals.) Counting calories and obsessive restriction of large food groups also has no place in a whole foods approach. Fat is not an enemy, and dairy is not off-limits. You just eat what your body was created to consume in its most natural (and digestible) form. You also modify if something doesn't seem to suit you for whatever reason—for example, if you are intolerant or allergic to any specific foods.

It's really remarkable how simple and logical this approach is yet many people walk around in a cloud of misleading nutrition information. When I introduce them to this concept, it's like a light bulb turns on. This isn't a shiny set of rules or a complicated list of "eats" and "eat-nots." It is logical, realistic, and unlimited in its potential for satisfaction.

Fun Food

I should reiterate here that perfection is not the goal. To eat only whole foods all the time would be really difficult, if not impossible. Yet, it's often helpful for people to have parameters or a goal in mind as they construct their grocery lists and meal plans, so this is the one I recommend:

> **Eat as many whole, natural foods as possible, and when you aren't eating whole foods, ditch the guilt and enjoy every bite.**

I once heard someone call foods that are more about *enjoyment* and *taste* than actual nourishment "fun foods." I love this term for many reasons. Many people use the term "junk foods" to describe these same foods, but I think that term is inappropriate. Merriam-Webster Dictionary defines "junk" as "something of poor quality" and "something of little meaning, worth, or significance."[7] Sure, some fun foods can be of lower quality or worth, but have you ever eaten a decadent dessert from a nice restaurant or a cake made with love by a family member? Surely you can't argue that those items are low quality or have no significance. You don't eat crème brulee and cupcakes for their nutrients, you eat them because they are fun to eat. They taste good. They are a treat. And guess what? That is okay!

Many people cannot believe their ears when I tell them that they are allowed to eat their favorite foods. They've been told for so long that those foods are bad and to be avoided. Not so! One of the first steps to making peace with your food and being able to eat in a healthy, sustainable way is learning how to enjoy those previously forbidden foods.

Sometimes I get asked, "What if I can't control myself and I eat too many of these foods?" People are often really concerned that they won't be able to handle themselves around the foods that previously were stumbling blocks. More times than not, these same people end up naturally cutting back on their fun food intake. When it isn't forbidden, they know it is always available, and thus it becomes a bit less desirable.

Plus, if you make feeling good a top priority in terms of what you choose to put into your body, you will end up choosing fewer of these foods. Whole foods are energizing, strengthening, and satisfying. On the other hand, fun foods tend to have the opposite effect, especially when eaten in excess. Have you ever eaten something to the point where you felt bloated, sluggish, mentally foggy, or even sick? With this new approach to eating, episodes like this will simply become less regular. Why would you eat something to the point of feeling ill if you know that you can have far less of it, enjoy every bite, and come back for more later if you really want it?

You may even find, as you go through this process, that your previously forbidden foods lose some of their luster for you. Some people discover they don't really like many of these foods at all. Many times, fun foods, especially those that are heavily processed, are designed to be eaten quickly and without much consideration in regard to their taste. For example, have you ever heard of someone getting out a bowl for a couple potato chips, then sitting at the table without distractions to savor every bite? Of course not! What is far more typical is the image of a person mindlessly munching from the bag, sitting on the couch, and watching TV. They aren't eating one chip at a time to really enjoy each; no, they are eating by the fistful, not thinking much about the flavor at all. When you start to really analyze the taste of some of your "favorite" fun foods, you may discover they aren't so wonderful after all.

On the other hand, giving yourself permission to have fun foods will allow you to enjoy those that you do choose to a greater extent. You may even become more discerning about the quality of fun foods you gravitate towards. Pre-packaged Chips-Ahoy! cookies start to taste pretty bland when you compare them to a freshly baked, warm cookie from your local bakery. No wonder you used to have to eat so many of them to get satisfied!

As a reminder, fill your meals with mostly whole, nutritious foods, and enjoy the occasional fun food as a treat. Fun foods are just that—fun—so enjoy them guilt-free. Just check in with how they make you feel and listen to your hunger and fullness signals, and they won't send you off course. More on this later in the   book.

4. WHEN WE WERE MEANT TO EAT

Q: When should you eat?

A: When you are hungry.

Boom! Pretty profound, right? The answer to when to eat is simple but can be difficult to execute. One reason for this is that we have lost touch with our hunger and fullness signals. We eat because the food is there, because it is the time of day that everyone is supposed to eat, or because we are bored, sad, lonely, and so on. Sometimes we do eat because we are hungry, but then comes the question of when to stop eating, and that is where we struggle. Fullness is a spectrum, and many people stop too far down it. We overstuff ourselves and are left feeling bloated, maybe even sick, and disappointed with ourselves yet again.

Hunger is the issue in question here, so we need to learn more about it, starting with the root: why do we get hungry? Hunger really serves an important purpose for us. It is the body's signal that it needs more fuel. Think of it as the arrow on your gas tank slowly getting closer to E. Just like the gas-tank arrow, hunger is gradual. It may start with subtle sensations—a slight emptiness to the stomach, or a churning or tightening.

Maybe you feel it in your mouth, and you start to salivate at the thought of food. Maybe you are having a hard time concentrating on your work.

It can eventually progress much further—closer to "E," if you will—where suddenly you feel lightheaded, your stomach actually hurts, and you feel ravenous. The key is not to let yourself get to this point because if you do, that will only mean trouble for you. You should eat something, even something small, when you first start noticing some hunger cues. Early on in the hunger process, you are better able to make rational decisions about what you will eat and how much. But, if you get overly hungry, a primal drive takes over and you will have a harder time choosing nutritious foods and not overeating.

Some people have a hard time eating breakfast because they are simply not hungry or because eating certain food or too much food will make them feel nauseated. Despite this, it is important to get some fuel in the body in the morning, even if it is something small. Experiment with what is the most palatable, energizes you, and keeps you satisfied the longest to determine what works best for you in the morning if you fall into this category.

What about your daily eating schedule? Most people follow the typical three meal schedule—breakfast, lunch, and dinner. This is usually how our lives are organized socially and professionally, so it makes sense to try to eat this way. I would argue, though, that for most people, only eating during those three meals is not frequent enough. Most people need snacks thrown into the mix to keep themselves from getting too hungry between meals.

Another alternative is to eat more frequent, smaller meals throughout the day. This works especially well if you have an atypical work schedule or stay home during the day.

Do what works for you in the moment where you find yourself. Experiment with it. See what keeps you feeling your best throughout the day.

Hunger is largely about stabilizing blood sugar. When you go too long between meals, your blood sugar plummets, setting off a whole string of undesirable consequences. When you eat lots of high-sugar foods, it will skyrocket, which is equally detrimental to how you feel as well as to your long-term health. The key is to stabilize your blood sugar, keeping it as even as possible throughout the day and minimizing dips and escalations. This will happen naturally if your diet is made up *mostly* of whole foods. Whole foods have fiber that slows down the digestion process and releases the sugars from the food more slowly into your bloodstream, which yields stabilization and a happy, satisfied you! You will likely feel hungry less frequently and, when it does hit, it will be subtler and less urgent.

Another important realization for most of my clients is that they are not going to starve. *Well, that's a given,* you may be thinking. But ask yourself this: When was the last time you ate more than you needed because you were afraid you would get hungry later? Why were you afraid of getting hungry at some unforeseen future moment? Would you not have access to food?

Most of the time, these fears are unfounded. Food is almost always available wherever you are, especially if you plan ahead with nutritious snacks. It is okay, even preferable, to stop eating if you are no longer hungry. Just tell yourself that food will still be available if you get hungry later, and you are allowed to eat when you are hungry again, even if it is within the hour of the last time you ate! Giving yourself permission to eat *whenever* you are hungry eliminates the need to overeat "just in case" you get hungry later.

On another note, a lot of people make a big deal about what

time at night to stop eating. While this advice has good intentions, it isn't something you need to be too rigid about. Lots of research shows that it doesn't matter what time you eat. In fact, for some people, eating a bedtime snack can actually be beneficial. Having something small can help stabilize your blood sugar through the night and keep you from waking up due to hunger. It can also make you feel less starved in the morning, which may help set you up for better eating choices through the rest of your day. The key here is to find what works for you and your body. If you do choose to have a little snack, have something small so that you don't put too much of a burden on your digestive system, which could lead to middle-of-the-night waking.

That being said, eating at night can be a trigger for people, leading them to eat foods they've been resisting during the day and over-consuming those foods as well. I often get a hankering for sweets in the evening hours, and I have to be careful to set myself up for success to stay in control of the situation. For me—this may be different than for you—but I know that I need to stay hydrated in the evening to avoid feeling "hungry," which is often really just dehydration. Sometimes I try drinking tea if I think I am hungry. If having something flavored is enough to satisfy me, then I wasn't hungry I was just bored and looking for a distraction. I love dark chocolate, so I often will treat myself to a piece of dark chocolate and eat it slowly, savoring every bite. Finally, if I am actually hungry during the late evening hours, I give myself full permission to eat something to satisfy that hunger, and you should too. Find what works for you and what serves your body best. We are all different, and our needs evolve!

5. HOW WE WERE MEANT TO EAT

As I launch into this section on *how* we were meant to eat, I want to say *again* that eating (and life for that matter) is not about perfection. It is about progress. The suggestions offered here are meant as guidelines, points for pondering, and goals to strive toward, even if you miss the mark sometimes. These recommendations probably aren't possible all the time but they are ideals that make up some of the ways in which we as humans were meant to eat. We are all works in progress, so just do your best, one day at a time.

Eat With Others

The first tenet of how we were meant to eat is this: Eating should be communal. We were meant to share meals around a table with people that we care about. Throughout history, eating has been a community event. The animal was hunted by a small group, brought home to the rest of the community, and cooked and shared amongst everyone. Our holiday traditions wouldn't be the same without a shared meal. Over meals, stories are told, political topics discussed, and plans for the future are made.

Shared meals are an important tradition in all societies, but unfortunately, the priority in our country has shifted from community to individualism in many ways. We went from living in multi-generational homes to living with just our nuclear family—if we have one, that is. Most people do not live close to their extended family and only see them during the holidays. Even our non-family communities tend to be restricted to the workplace, the place of worship on Sundays, and maybe the occasional social gathering.

We need to bring the community table back. Ideally, we would share many more eating experiences with people we care about. Having friends and family over for dinner may seem like a lot of work, but it doesn't have to be, when the focus is not on impressing everyone with some fancy meal, but rather on enjoying the company of loved ones. Follow this wise saying: KISS—Keep It Simple Stupid. Cook something simple that you already know your family enjoys, and don't get hung up on the details or clean up. Better yet, use disposable dishes and utensils if that will help you to enjoy your time more!

Beyond hosting for others, if you live with people—family or roommates—make an attempt to eat as many meals as possible together. You will see your relationships grow and your meals become more satisfying.

Prior to becoming a health coach and author, I was a high-school teacher, which forced me to be out the door before my husband was even out of bed. I often grabbed whatever I could get my hands on for breakfast and ate quickly as I finished up my makeup or even as I drove to work. It was not a good way to start my day—just another thing to check off my list as I ran out the door. Now, we eat together, our daughter included, every morning. It isn't a long meal, but I love that we get to start our mornings together, and I love the example we are setting for our little girl.

If you eat at work, you also have an opportunity to develop

community with your coworkers over a meal. Most workplaces have some sort of break room where you can choose to eat. If you have shared lunch breaks, eating as a group can be a nice change of pace from the office humdrum. Lunch is an opportunity to talk about things besides work and to get to know your coworkers in a new light. Taking these opportunities when you can will likely lead to a more satisfying work life and better relationships with your coworkers.

Eat at the Table

Eating with others is important, but it is equally important to consider *where* you eat. We are a nation that eats on the go—in our cars, at our desks, standing in the kitchen, at our kids' soccer games, and in front of the TV. The truth is, we were meant to eat sitting down, at the table.

It would be hard to argue that you enjoy your rushed meal in the car as you swerve through traffic more than one where you sit down at the table to eat. You can hardly pay attention to the road in front of you and the cars around you, let alone the taste of the sandwich you are hastily eating. Plus, if you eat on-the-go, you are less likely to listen to your hunger and fullness signals, and you are more likely to overeat.

I have a client who had a hard time with mindlessly snacking. Watching TV went hand-in-hand with munching on something for her. To combat this, I told her she could still watch TV and have her snack, but she had to be sitting at her kitchen table (where she can still see the TV) while she ate. This resulted in less snacking on her part because the eating became less of a habit. She only got up to get a snack if she was hungry, and stopped when she was full because she wanted to go back and sit on the comfy couch to watch the TV.

Be Mindful

If I were to summarize *how* to eat, I would be left with two words—*mindful eating*. Mindful eating is the art of eating food in a way that brings your entire awareness to the experience. You notice your hunger, choose foods that will best satisfy your needs, eat them in a fully present state, and stop when you are no longer hungry.

Being still, minimizing distractions, and focusing on the meal allows you to experience your food with all of your senses, an important aspect of mindful eating. This kind of approach is shown to not only bring more pleasure to the eating experience, but also will help you to be aware of your hunger and fullness so you are less likely to overeat.

Becoming a mindful eater is like reconnecting with your toddler self—before your relationship with food became flawed. A toddler will observe a new food. She turns it around and around in her hands, both to feel its texture and to look at it from every angle. She then brings it to her nose and smells it, usually pulling it away to ponder the odor she just smelled. If she decides to continue on, she may touch it to her tongue for the smallest of tastes. She rolls her tongue around in her mouth, allowing the taste to linger a while longer. If she decides she likes what she has tasted, or at a minimum is curious about what she has tasted and wants to explore further, she will take a bite.

Have you ever noticed how slowly a small child eats? For many parents, it is *painstakingly* slow. *Don't you know we've got somewhere to be?* The truth is, these kids are acting on their natural inclinations. We have just lost touch with ours as adults.

Small children, especially before their parents begin manipulating their eating patterns, are mindful eaters. They eat with all of their senses, and they listen to their hunger and fullness signals. As many parents know, it is pretty tough to get a child to eat when they are no longer hungry. Cue the airplane spoon. *Here comes the airplane. Vrooooom!* Many well-meaning parents use this kind of technique, but the result is that their child becomes more and more separated from the naturally mindful eater that they were born as. They are inadvertently recruiting them to become members of the Clean Plate Club. Ring a bell?

We were all mindful eaters once. We just need to go back to that. A large portion of this book is devoted to helping you rediscover those original habits and develop a skillset that will benefit you for the rest of your life. Read on for practical ways to incorporate mindful eating into your life.

Make Gratitude Part of Your Meals

All of the running around from one thing to the next not only makes it difficult for us to eat mindfully but also doesn't leave any time for gratitude. Gratitude is the state of being thankful and showing appreciation for the things you have been given. Practicing gratitude makes people happier and more compassionate, and also improves sleep. It even has been shown to strengthen your immune system!

There has been some interesting scientific research done regarding the effects of gratitude. Dr. Robert A. Emmons of the University of California, Davis and Dr. Michael E. McCullough of the University of Miami did a study looking at this very topic. For the study, they separated participants into three groups. All three of the groups kept "journals" where they wrote a few sentences each week.

The first group wrote down things for which they were grateful; the second wrote down things that happened that bothered or upset them; and the third group wrote down events that stuck out to them, but didn't comment on whether they were good or bad. They wrote about these events very matter-of-factly.

As a result of the study, the first group (the one that expressed gratitude) displayed more optimism, and they were happier with their lives. The researchers even noticed that this group spent more time being physically active and required fewer doctor visits. Being grateful makes you not only emotionally healthier but also physically healthier![8]

Gratitude doesn't have to be reserved for the big moments in life, either. Of course it is natural to be grateful for certain things—the birth of a child, a marriage, graduation, promotion, overcoming life-threatening illness, etc.—but you can also express gratitude throughout the day, even if nothing monumental happens. In fact, stretching yourself a bit to be thankful for the little things will, over time, cause a mental shift where you are more appreciative of the world around you.

There are many ways to practice gratitude. One example is keeping a gratitude journal like subjects in the above study did. You can also pray or simply say "thank you" to someone who has done something kind for you. As it relates to eating—the topic of this book—I would like to suggest incorporating gratitude into your routine at meals.

The most obvious way to do this is to pause before your meal, and say a prayer or a few words about what you are grateful for in that meal or what you are grateful for from that day so far. Cultivating an attitude of gratitude will remind you that there are blessings that come into our lives that are beyond us. Remembering those blessings and not taking them for granted will help you to be steadier during life's ups and downs. Sometimes it is all too easy to focus on the bad, forgetting the good, when really we have so much to be thankful for. Making this a practice—and yes, it takes practice—will yield many positive results.

In addition to making you happier and more loving and compassionate, improving your sleep and immune function, and getting you moving more, practicing gratitude may help you eat more healthfully. The act of pausing for a moment before you dig in to your plate and focusing your thoughts is very centering. It helps you tune in to what is going on inside of you. Maybe even try a couple deep breaths at this time, and think about your intention for the meal, what you are eating, how you will eat it, and when you will stop. You may find yourself even more capable of listening to your body, eating more of what will nourish you, and stopping before you go too far.

6. WHAT FOOD IS NOT MEANT TO BE

We've just spent the last few sections discussing what food is meant to be and how it is meant to be used. It is meant as nourishment for our minds, bodies, and souls. We are meant to use it to nutritionally sustain ourselves, to build community with those we care about, and to bring pleasure into our lives. We should be grateful for all of our blessings in life, including the foods we consume everyday.

It is a sad truth for many that food is a major pain point in their lives. Dieting is just one manifestation of an unhealthy relationship with food. For some, food is a substitute for love and companionship. For others, it serves as an escape or distraction from their stressful lives. Lastly, food can be used as reward or punishment.

All of these uses represent unhealthy, broken relationships with food. They can develop quickly or over a span of many years, but many begin in childhood as the result of something that has happened or something that we learned from our parents. We have already discussed how well-meaning parents often push their kids to eat even when they don't want to, one of the first instances through which these little ones learn to ignore their bodies' innate signals. Parents have a huge impact on how their children's relationships with food develop—for better or worse.

We are each, to some degree, a product of our childhood. With regards to food and eating, you probably came away with a mixed bag. There were likely some skills or habits that your parents passed on that have been helpful, but there are also probably some that are not. Maybe even some of the things your parents did had a *really* negative impact on your relationship with food.

Maybe your parents gave you treats whenever you were hurt or something bad happened. You may have learned to associate emotional or physical pain with the need for something sweet. Maybe your parents had a tumultuous relationship, where they were always fighting. You may have chosen to block out their screams by digging into a bag of chips. It's also possible that you were raised in a household where you never felt good enough. Every time that you would do something wrong, your favorite foods would be taken away as punishment. Maybe you were forced to clean your plate even if you were no longer hungry. On the other hand, maybe food was used as a carrot dangling on a stick. If you behaved well, you would be given some sort of treat. And if you didn't, you could forget it.

There are all kinds of potential long-term problems associated with all of these situations. If it is frequent enough, being given sweets when you are sad or hurt or as a reward for good behavior can lead to an association between a sugary treat and those emotions. *Things aren't going well at work—I need cake! I'm so upset with my husband—bring on the cookies!* Even the positive moments can bring about the need to eat. *I finally finished that assignment—I deserve to treat myself!*

If you regularly turned to food as a means of escape or distraction, you will likely continue that behavior every time a new stressor comes into your life. *I can't handle caring for my aging parents—I'm going to eat and forget about it for a bit! I don't know how we will make our payments this month—forget it, I need some pizza! My family and job responsibilities are overwhelming—I deserve a treat!*

If food has been a punishment for you, you may self-punish if you feel guilty about something bad or undeserving of something good coming into your life. Self-sabotage is something people do in this situation, and they often use food to do it. Maybe things are going well in one area of your life, so you feel like you need to do something as to not jinx it. You may overeat to the point of being uncomfortable as a way to bring balance back. As illogical as this may sound to some, this is a very common occurrence with people who regularly use food as a punishment or reward.

With all of these examples, food is being used for a reason. In one way or another, it is serving the person that is using it, and it is momentarily effective. It makes them feel good when they feel bad or are in need of a reward, it distracts when the stress of life is overwhelming, and it can even make them feel bad if they want to punish themselves.

The problem is, after the pizza is polished off or the ice cream carton is empty, whatever situation or feeling triggered the binge is still there. You haven't really dealt with the root cause, and now, to add insult to injury, you are stuffed and uncomfortable and further upset with yourself for overdoing it with the food. The problem suddenly magnifies, and if you aren't equipped with the skills to handle it, you are likely going to resort to your tried-and-true method—using food to deal (or really, not deal) with it.

This is not your fault or a reflection of your character flaws. These are habits that are formed early in life, are largely unavoidable, and are difficult to break. Luckily for you, the rest of this book is about making right your relationship with food. Whether you suffer from some of the deeper emotional eating issues described above or you have just been a casual dieter who is tired of the endless cycle of that particular path, there are answers for you ahead. Get ready to change your eating, and thus change your life, forever.

PART TWO:
GET YOUR HEAD ON STRAIGHT

7. THE MENTAL GAME

In the previous section, I demonstrated why dieting is the wrong means to weight loss and, probably more importantly, can be a leading contributor to an unhealthy relationship with food. I then went on to outline what, when, and how we were meant to eat. Lastly, I discussed the ways that we were *not* meant to use food.

The previous section was philosophical in nature. These next two sections are more practical—the "how-to" of this book. There are lots of steps and suggestions presented here, and my recommendation is that you pick and choose what you think will be most helpful in your situation. Some things I discuss will be especially helpful for certain people but maybe not for others, and some would be good for everyone to put into practice. We are all different, so experiment and find what feels appropriate for you.

Part Two focuses on the internal changes that have to occur in order to fix your relationship with food. Simply changing a few behaviors will not result in a healthy relationship with food that is sustainable and real. You have to do the mental work first. The suggestions outlined here may take quite a bit of time for you to get through. It will take as long as it takes, but remember, it is your health and wellbeing at stake. Do not rush through the process.

What you have been doing hasn't been working, and we've discussed the reasons why. One of the biggest reasons is that there are deeper food issues at play that you have probably never addressed. This is the mental part of the equation—the part that requires some serious attention before we even begin to address the eating. It's also the part that diets don't address. With a diet, you are given a list of "eats" and "eat-nots," maybe some explanation for the list, and usually some testimonials to get you revved up, but you are never encouraged to dig deep to make the mental shifts necessary to really *heal*. That's the work we will begin with—the nuts and bolts of what has held you back and what can propel you forward. The healing starts from within.

There is no one correct path through this. You may also uncover some difficult and painful feelings and memories along the way. This is a necessary part of healing, but if you find that this happens for you, you may want to consider getting additional support from a health coach, therapist, doctor, or other wellness professional.

A Note About Weight

In order to be successful, you need to decide here and now to detach yourself from the goal of weight loss. *WHAT?!*—you are probably thinking—*That's the whole reason I bought this book!* Look, I am not saying that you *won't* lose weight. In fact, it is very likely that you will. The thing is, in order to be successful, you have to replace the goal of weight loss with the goal of a healthy relationship with food. When that is in place, when you are eating in a way that is intuitive and respectful of *all* of your needs—psychological, spiritual, and physical—your body will naturally move towards your healthy weight.

Are you ready for the next, potentially disappointing truth? You and your body may have different ideas about what your healthy weight set point actually is. It may not be the number you have been longing for all of these years and potentially is higher than what you think.

But what about BMI? Isn't BMI a good indicator of what my healthy weight range is? Not really, according to the latest science. BMI is an incomplete assessment. It only takes into account your height and weight to give you a number that supposedly tells you if you are healthy or not. This is problematic for a couple of reasons. First, it doesn't take any consideration for fat versus muscle in your total weight. Muscle weighs more than fat, yet it would be hard to argue that a toned athlete is unhealthy, even if he or she falls into the overweight category. In fact, NFL quarterback Tom Brady is an excellent example of this. At 6 feet 4 inches and 225 pounds, he has a BMI of 27.4, which puts him right in the middle of the overweight range. Is he unhealthy then? Quite the contrary! He is the picture of good health.

In addition, BMI fails to look at types of fat and where that fat is stored on the body. For example, we all have some amount of fat under our skin, called subcutaneous fat. This is the fat that you have on the fleshy parts of your body—your thighs, butt, and the part that you can pinch on your arms. Many scientists and doctors don't think that this particular type of fat causes health problems.

Rather, it is the belly fat, also known as visceral fat, which wraps around your organs, that is the real troublemaker. Visceral fat, apart from expanding our waistlines, also undermines our health in a number of ways. First, it releases certain hormones and toxins that mess with the body's normal functioning. It makes us more likely to become insulin resistant, thus potentially leading to diabetes. In addition, it is a risk factor for heart disease and certain cancers, and even has been linked to dementia! Some people that are not considered obese according to their BMI may in fact have high levels of visceral fat, putting them at risk for all these health issues.

The point is that BMI—currently the most widely accepted indicator of a healthy weight range—is insufficient. So, what is your healthy weight? It's truly unique to the individual. You can find out, though, by following the steps I present in this book to heal your relationship with food and begin eating the way you were meant to eat. If you are not at your healthy weight already, which you probably aren't if your relationship with food is broken, your body will begin readjusting. You will notice your body changing as you move towards your unique set point. Clothes may loosen and friends may make comments about how you look like you've lost weight. Great—but remember that WEIGHT LOSS IS NOT YOUR GOAL. Your goal and mantra moving forward is this:

I am on a journey to mend my broken relationship with food so that I can live a healthy and happy life.

If weight loss is a result of that journey, so be it, but remember that weight loss is secondary. Life is so much more than a number on a scale. You could push yourself lower than your healthy weight set point, but at what cost? Continuing to restrict and starve and miss out and obsess about food? You can't live your life chasing some distant, unrealistic dream body you used to have, your friend has, or some celebrity has.

The trade-off is freedom and *real* health and wellness. You will never again have to be a slave to the scale or constantly worried about your appearance. Guilt will be a thing of the past, and you will enjoy eating and living at a new level.

This may seem like some kind of fantasy. *Easier said than*

done, right? You're right. It *is* easier said than done, but I am up for the challenge of walking you through the steps to get there if you are willing to do the work. Body acceptance is a necessary component of healthy living and eating, and through reading this book, you will do the work of starting to love your body enough to treat it gently, with kind actions and thoughts. This is all ahead in the coming chapters. For now, I have one question for you:

Are you ready?

It will likely be challenging work, but it will be worth it. You have run from these issues for too long. How has that helped you? You are likely even worse off than you were a few years ago. "Hitting rock bottom" has all kinds of negative connotations, but what if this is your "rock bottom"? What if the only way to go is up? What if this is your moment, your turning point that you can look back on years from now and say, "That is when I decided to change my life!"

Do you want it? Do you want to be free from food? Do you want to be able to eat like a normal person, enjoying both nutritious and delicious foods without obsessing, shaming, and beating yourself up? Do you want to find your healthy weight that is unique to your beautiful body and maintain it with ease?

If you answered "yes" to the questions above, then buckle up. It's going to be a bumpy, exciting, and life-changing ride.

8. DISCOVER YOUR "WHY"

I am going to ask you a question that, at first glance, may seem very simple. Why are you on this journey? In other words, why do you want to change and embrace a new, healthy relationship with food?

Maybe your answer is like many of my clients' when they first come to see me. "I want to lose weight," or *slightly* better, "I want to get healthy." Okay, but *why*?

You see, the above answers aren't the real reason why you are seeking a change in your life. They are just the surface answer you've been giving for many years. You probably don't even know that it is a surface answer. *Isn't that the reason most everyone gives for changing the way they eat?* Yes, but need I remind you how that's working out for most people? Not too well.

So, maybe you initially said that you want to "get healthy." That's a fine start, but it isn't the real reason. *Why* do you want to get healthy? Have you ever really thought about it before? Maybe you want to "get healthy" for one or a combination of any of the following reasons:

- You are tired of feeling uncomfortable in your body

- You want more energy to play with your kids or do activities you used to love
- You have a family history of lifestyle diseases and don't want to get sick
- You want more confidence
- You have a responsibility to be a role model in your family

Come up with your own "why" list. Feel free to be inspired by some of the reasons mentioned above. Why are you reading this book? What are you hoping to get from it? How are you hoping your life changes? Go write your list. No, seriously, go now! This book will still be waiting when you get back.

Discover Your "Why": The Letter

Now that you have your list, you are now going to write a letter to yourself about why you want to change. This will be your Intention Letter. This may sound corny, but it can be a very effective way of getting your thoughts out, analyzing them, and then turning them into action.

You should now look at your list as an outline for your letter. In addition to the "why" statements you have on your list, consider the following questions as you write your letter:

- What do you hope to achieve?
- What do you want to change about your life now?
- How would life be different if you achieved your goals?
- How would you feel?
- How would others perceive you?
- Whose life could you positively impact?

Sometimes, it is easier for us to convey our hopes and dreams for our loved ones more than our hopes and dreams for ourselves. Mothers, especially, have this dilemma. They are always worried about the well-being and the future of their children, and they often neglect their own needs.

This can actually be a helpful lens for taking a look at your own life and choices. If you are having trouble with writing this letter to yourself, especially if you are having a hard time finding a gentle, loving voice to write it in, consider looking at it as if you were looking at someone you love very dearly, such as a child.

- How do you want your loved ones to relate with food?
- What kinds of choices do you hope that they make?
- How would you want their relationship with food to differ from yours?
- Why?

This can help you flesh out some of your thoughts as you write this letter to yourself. If you want these things for those closest to you, shouldn't you also want the same things for yourself? We always want the best for those that we love. We should start seeking the same for ourselves.

Once you have finished your Intention Letter, put it somewhere safe and accessible. It should be somewhere that you can pull it out regularly to read and remind yourself of your goals and your reasons behind those goals. When you find yourself losing motivation or questioning the path you are on, pull this out and read it.

You have now examined the reason why you are on this journey. Now we are going to take a look at some of the mental obstacles that may be in your path.

9. YOUR BELIEFS ARE THE PROBLEM

Whether you believe you can do a thing or not, you are right.

-- Henry Ford

All of the experiences in your life affect who you are, what you believe about yourself, and how you act according to those beliefs. A major stumbling block to weight loss is the beliefs we hold about ourselves. The beliefs you hold onto or the stories you tell yourself can become excuses to use food inappropriately and a wall to any progress. Some examples of beliefs that can do this to you are:

I have no self-control.

I am ugly.

I hate vegetables.

I don't deserve love or companionship.

I'm not as good/beautiful/intelligent/funny as...

I am never going to lose weight.

These thoughts are common among people who have a

broken relationship with food and eating. The thing is, they are NOT *truths*; they are *beliefs*, and ill-conceived beliefs at that. Take any one of them and ask yourself, "How do I know this to be true?" For example you could ask, "How do I know I am never going to lose weight?" Can you really KNOW this to be true? Sure, maybe you haven't been successful with weight loss in the past, but how do you KNOW you never will in the future? You can't!

Take any of the above beliefs and if you think about them enough, you will see that you cannot know any of them to be 100-percent irrefutably true. You believe you hate vegetables? Are you sure? Have you tried all of them? Have you experimented with how you prepare them?

I have had clients that thought that they hated vegetables. Once we dug a little deeper, though, they've revealed that their only experiences with vegetables were the canned vegetables they grew up being forced to eat by their parents. Yuck! I love many vegetables, but I would hate them too if that had been my experience! After we discussed a variety of preparation methods and I encouraged them to experiment with some new vegetables, they all have found that there are some that they actually *like* and can prepare at home! Belief changed!

So how do you do this for yourself? First, get out a piece of paper or a notebook and make a list of all the beliefs you hold that you think have had an affect on your relationship with food. Feel free to borrow from the example list above if any of those ring true, but also add others that you think apply to your situation. Next, spend time examining each item on your Beliefs List. Really think about it. Ask yourself:

- Is this true?
- Am I 100-percent sure?
- How can I KNOW it is true?

At this point, you probably have discovered that they are not truths, but beliefs. Now, you need to find counterarguments against each of these beliefs. Look back at your life and see if there have been any events that prove that these beliefs aren't true. It's interesting—when we believe something, we often seek out things that support our beliefs and actively ignore things that may cast doubt on them. It's time to stop that. You need to step back from the belief and take a neutral perspective. Ask yourself these questions:

- When in my life has this belief not been true?
- When have I chosen to ignore or forget situations that didn't reinforce my beliefs?
- Who has told me that some of these beliefs are not true?
- Are there ways that I can prove them to be false, or at least not true all of the time?

Some of these beliefs may be really ingrained after being reinforced by years of experiences. It is possible that you really think that these are true for you. But even if a belief is true, does it have to be? Can it change? What if it could? Maybe your past makes it almost impossible not to believe, but one way to know that they are not TRUE is that you cannot look into the future and know for certain that they will continue being true.

I recommend writing out belief counterargument statements on a separate sheet of paper from your Beliefs List. This will be your Truths List. For example, if you had written, "I have no self-control," on your Beliefs List, and you remembered a time when you refrained from dessert because you were already too full, then you would put, "I showed self-control last week when I didn't eat that cheesecake after dinner," on your Truths List. These statements should be as action-based and factual as possible. Do your best to avoid making judgment statements, such as "I did a *good* job last week when I didn't eat that cheesecake." They should be neutral statements.

Once you have taken a hard look at your beliefs and proven that they are not true, it's time to let them go. Maybe you want to tear your Beliefs List up and throw it into the trash. For some people, going as far as to burn their list can be very meaningful. Do whatever sounds good, cathartic, and appropriate for you.

Be careful of the temptation to hold onto your Beliefs List. You may be thinking that you'd like to have it to look back at later, but why? Those beliefs aren't true anyway! You just proved it with all your counterarguments. You have your Truths List now, and truths are so much more valuable than false beliefs. Holding onto those beliefs to periodically read is just bringing things up that didn't ever help you in the first place. They make you feel bad about yourself and they trap you, holding you back from positive change. It is time to let go of the beliefs that don't serve you, for good.

10. MAKE PEACE WITH YOUR BODY

It's time for some real talk. Whether you like it or not, you were only given one body for this lifetime, so it's time to make peace with it and start treating it better. We have all been there, staring at a sibling, a friend, or the cover of a magazine and thinking, "I wish I had *that*!" All of a sudden, any positive thoughts we had about ourselves go out the window, only to be replaced with ugly thoughts of jealousy and self-deprecation.

I have been there! My first memory of body insecurity is of when my grandfather mentioned in an off-hand way that my thighs were getting "fat." I think I was six or seven years old, and I can very clearly remember staring in the full-length mirror in my parents' room regularly after that, thinking, "Are my legs fat? They must be if he said so!" I had never felt bad about my body before that.

In fifth grade, my teacher had us do an exercise that was meant to build each other up. We were each assigned a random letter of the alphabet and were told to come up with a word that started with that letter to describe another person in the class. The boy that was supposed to describe me was given "J," and his word for me that he shared with the entire class—"Jenny Craig."

I have a sister who was taller and thinner than I was while growing up, and I played sports where the majority of my teammates weighed less than I did. In college I joined a sorority that was teeming with size-zeros and flat tummies. I let many of those things affect how I thought about myself. It took a lot of hard work to get over those comparisons and find peace with the body I had, but I got there eventually. I want that for you, too.

The truth is that we are all built differently. I will NEVER look like a Victoria's Secret model or an Olympic athlete, and I have come to terms with that being OKAY. In fact, I have even gotten to the point where I am thankful for my body and the unique things about it that make me *me*. As the old adage goes, "Variety is the spice of life!" If everyone looked and behaved the same, this place would be incredibly boring. Beauty is just one characteristic that a person may have, and it is a very subjective one at that. There is so much more to a person that gives them worth.

Have you ever considered that being beautiful (according to society's standards) may not even be desirable? I know, you probably think I'm crazy for even bringing up this notion, but it is something to think about. There are definitely challenges that exceptionally "beautiful" people face that other people don't.

For one, the characteristic most people associate with them is their beauty, not their intelligence, wit, creativity, etc. Because external forces are constantly reinforcing their appearance and not much else, they may have a hard time believing in themselves in other areas of their lives. You see this all the time where people end up craving this kind of attention, living off of it, because they get their sense of self-worth from external forces, not from within.

Often, beautiful people find that doors (figuratively) open more readily for them. They get more dates, job opportunities, and attention. Because of this, they are less likely to hone skills that help them in these situations. They simply don't need them. They can just show their pretty face, flash a million-dollar smile, and they get what they want. Problems arise when something does come up in which they can't get by on looks alone—they simply do not know what to do.

Another problem with being exceptionally beautiful is its social consequences. While they may have no problem getting romantic attention, friends may be harder to come by. Resentment brews when all the attention goes to one particular person every time they enter the room, and, because of this, women tend to shy away from other women whom they perceive to be much more attractive than they are.

Lastly, beauty is fleeting. Everyone, no matter how beautiful they are, will age. They will get wrinkles and probably gain weight. What will they do then if all they had before was their appearance? Aging tends to be much harder on these people, since so much of their self-worth and identity is tied up in how they look.

I share this perspective not to disparage good-looking people, but rather to offer another point of view. We all have our own stories and our own struggles, no matter how perfect someone's life seems on the outside.

I want you to stop chasing some unrealistic, and potentially unhealthy, ideal. I also want you to stop berating yourself for your "failure" to get the body of your dreams. I'm going to make a statement that is sure to get some eye rolls: Your body is an amazing—and, yes, truly beautiful—work of art! Okay, cue the sarcastic, "Yeah, right." Look, it's unlikely you are ready to make that leap just yet, but you absolutely can start appreciating your unique body in ways you never have before.

Consider this: Your heart pumps all day every day and brings blood to all of your vital organs. Your lungs bring in oxygen and expel carbon dioxide to feed every cell in your body. Your skin keeps your internal organs protected from outside infection. Your digestive system handles everything you put in your mouth—quite a feat sometimes! All of these are things that your wonderful body does for you without you giving it a second thought.

Beyond the internal, subconscious functioning of your body, there are things that your body does for you that are truly remarkable as well. You have eyes that give you a window into the beauty of the world around you, legs that propel you forward and backwards, and hips that sway to music.

So, what about your appearance? You may not be thrilled with what you've got, but hopefully there are some features that you are at least okay with, maybe that you even like! Maybe you don't love your stomach, but what about your eyes, hair, nose or lips? Think outside the box a bit. Have you ever thought about the appearance of your hands, ankles, neck, and toes? Can you appreciate some of those things about yourself?

Let's do another writing exercise. At the top of the paper, write, "I am Uniquely Beautiful." Now spend some time answering the following questions:

- What energizes or excites you?
- What are you passionate about?
- What are the things that make you unique?
- What do you have to offer the world?
- What is your purpose in life?
- What do you like about yourself?
- What do you like specifically about your body?
- What have others complimented you on before?
- What would other people say are your best features?

- What do you say are your best features?
- How can you highlight your best features?

Allow yourself to find your unique beauty externally and internally. Many people have a hard time expressing the things they like about themselves because they think it makes them look arrogant. But there is a difference between arrogance and respect. Respect yourself and your body for what it has to offer you and those around you. You are special and beautiful.

LINDSAY REINHOLT

11. SURROUND YOURSELF WITH POSITIVE MESSAGES

One of the main reasons why so many people have body image issues has to do with the media that surrounds us. We are constantly under attack, being told we are not good enough as we are, and we should be doing something to get skinnier. Morning news shows do stories about weight loss techniques, and magazine covers make ridiculous promises, like "2 Weeks to Bikini-Ready!"

Even the social media we *choose* to consume can do more harm than good. Following certain people on Instagram, Twitter, Snapchat or Facebook can expose you to images or ideas that make you feel bad about yourself. For example, that "fitness model" on Instagram probably isn't very motivating; she probably just makes you feel terrible by comparison every time she posts an image of her six-pack.

It is probably time for you to take a hard look at what you choose to consume in the media. Some things are unavoidable. You can't go to the grocery store without encountering all kinds of magazines with headlines about weight loss and beautiful celebrities, but you can choose not to look at them and definitely not to buy any. You can also change your voluntary media habits. Unfollow accounts that bring up negative emotions. Feeling like a failure is not helpful and blocks change, so only surround yourself with positive messages that inspire you rather than tear you down.

The media is a powerful influence, but it isn't the only place we receive messages about our bodies and weight. The people in our lives—our friends, family members, and coworkers—can unknowingly add to the problem.

Have you ever noticed how women *love* to talk badly about themselves to each other? "Ugh, I feel so fat!" "My skin looks horrible lately." "After the holidays, I've got to start a diet." And on and on it goes. As twisted as it may be, it does function as a sort of bonding ritual. Let's all talk about our inadequacies to show that we are all insecure, *together*!

As hard as it may be, it is best not to participate in these types of situations. It's fascinating, once you start paying attention, how frequently these conversations come up and how natural it is to join in. Do your best to start training yourself to see them coming and practice some strategies for bowing out. Excuse yourself to the bathroom, compliment someone else instead of focusing negatively on yourself, or even share with the group that you are working on ridding yourself of negative self-talk. Be prepared for some backlash, though. People can be very defensive in these moments because they reveal their own shortcomings. Read the situation and choose your actions accordingly. Above all, be compassionate and avoid passing judgment. We are all living our own story and struggling with our own junk.

When women do participate in this kind of behavior, they are not only tearing themselves down and proclaiming to themselves and the world, "I am not good enough!" but they are also condoning the platform on which others can follow suit. The point is, even if it is difficult or unnatural at first, refusing to participate in this kind of self-demoralizing talk is a step towards a higher level of self-acceptance and respect for *everyone*.

12. BANISH GUILT

Guilt is a convoluted emotion. As a child if you did something wrong, you were expected to feel guilty afterward. Guilt is almost considered a virtuous behavior. It demonstrates that you know you did something wrong and you feel bad about it. Some people feel guilt more readily than others, and people that don't feel guilty after doing something that others perceive as morally wrong are viewed as corrupt, uncompassionate people.

On the other hand, it is well recognized that guilt can have a hugely negative impact on the person feeling it, especially when it's not correctly addressed. "Guilt can eat you alive" is a common saying for a reason. Maybe you have even experienced it to a certain degree. Have you ever done something that you felt so guilty about that it tore you up inside? You probably couldn't think about much anything else at the time. When someone lets guilt slowly consume them, they feel more and more like a failure and cannot take steps to remedy the situation and move on.

When eating food is the source of our guilt, it traps us. It confirms our negative beliefs about ourselves and casts doubt on progress we've made. It keeps us stuck in a place where we dwell on past choices and we can't move on toward our goals. Guilt has no place in a healthy relationship with food.

The thing is, it is just food. There is nothing righteous about it, and conversely, there is nothing sinful about it. You are not harming anyone else by eating something versus not eating something, and, believe it or not, one meal, one day, even one week of eating more indulgent food will not be the end of you. Your wellness is built on more than just your eating choices, and it is all of your eating choices added up over a longer period of time that affect your wellbeing, not one Thanksgiving dinner or a weeklong trip to Mexico.

No matter what you choose to eat, you can learn from it and use it to better inform your future choices, rather than obsessing over it and letting it own you. You need to own *it!* You cannot go back and change it anyway. What's done is done. You made the choice, and it must have served you in some way in that moment.

Finding ways to reframe eating behaviors you naturally start feeling guilty about is an important habit to cultivate when banishing guilt. When you have one too many cookies as your bedtime treat, refrain from the negative self-talk. Instead of, "Well, I did it again! I ate all those cookies because I'm fat and I will never lose weight and I am a failure!" try, "Wow, those cookies were delicious, but I'm not sure that I needed all six. I wonder why I ate so many?"

Explore *why* you made the choice you made and use that information to make new choices down the road. Become an observer of your own habits. With the cookie example, maybe consider the possibility that you hadn't eaten enough for dinner, and you let yourself get overly hungry before you got a snack. Or maybe you had restricted sweets all day, and your craving eventually got the best of you, and you overindulged then at night. Maybe you are stressed at home or work and eating cookies was your way of comforting yourself in that moment.

Think about the possible reasons and brainstorm some strategies to prevent it from happening again down the road. Some obvious things to try would be eating a more filling dinner, having some sweet things sprinkled throughout the day to satisfy that craving before it gets out of control, and using alternative coping mechanisms for dealing with your stress. Let go of the guilt, learn, and move on better equipped to handle similar situations in the future.

LINDSAY REINHOLT

13. GET EDUCATED

One of the most powerful tools in your arsenal to nurture a healthy relationship with food is information. Diet is one of the leading contributors to obesity and all of its related health conditions, so although I am against "Do Not Eat" lists, I do recognize that the foods you choose to eat *do* matter. As mentioned previously, once-in-awhile fun foods *do not* ruin your health, but the sum of all of your food choices over time *does* have an impact.

At the most basic level, eating whole foods is the best way to go. Most health experts agree, eating food in its natural form is superior to eating processed food. Where you will find opposing sides is in the question of macronutrients (i.e. what is the best proportion of fat to protein to carbohydrate), whether dairy or other animal products are suitable for human consumption, and other more specific issues. I am not saying that these aren't topics worthy of discussion, but I don't think you need to get too hung up on these issues, especially if it is overwhelming to you. Nutrition is an evolving science, and there is a lot about it that we don't know.

That being said, despite the conflicting arguments, I do believe it is valuable to be informed, especially on the issues that you find interesting in the world of health and food. For many people, ignorance is bliss. It is easy to go on eating a certain way if you do not know the effects of those foods on your body. Understanding the realities of your food choices can be a powerful motivating factor to continue fueling your body with the best foods for it.

We've already discussed the overload of information out there on this topic, so it can be intimidating knowing where to begin. Start by paying more attention to the media to see if experts with whom you connect are featured or interviewed. Get recommendations from friends and family that are interested in this topic as well. Finding people and experts that you trust is important, but remember to seek information that resonates with you and your unique body and lifestyle.

A word of caution: Avoid diet books that have strict food rules or promote the sole goal of weight loss. This is the very thing you are trying to avoid. Remember, we have already learned that diets don't help us lose weight but rather may cause weight gain in addition to all kinds of other negative outcomes, physical and psychological. Look for books that are informative and interesting, but not restrictive.

It is also important to read books by authors that obviously *love* food. This isn't a hard thing to figure out. If the language of the book vilifies food, making it seem like a force to fight against, then the author is not someone who is promoting love for food. Remember, you are seeking a healthy *relationship* with food and relationships are built on trust, quality time, and love. Look for language that demonstrates this.

14. GOAL-SETTING

In order to be successful, you need to be clear on your goals. Getting really clear may take some time, but it will give you direction and a path to move forward to actually accomplishing them. In addition, goals provide focus to guide you and increase your productivity and commitment. Plus, goal-setting is a great boost to your self-esteem. It feels really good when you set goals and go on to accomplish them!

Maybe it is true that "there are no bad questions," but there can definitely be bad goals. The type of goals that you set really does make a difference. So what kinds of goals work the best? Well, first, goals that are thoughtfully written out are more likely to stick. Beyond that, your goals should be S.M.A.R.T. – Specific, Measurable, Attainable, Realistic, and Timely. Let's break that down a bit further.

S – Specific

A goal should be specific in that it should be precise and exact. The goal "I want to be healthy" is pretty vague. "Healthy" can mean all sorts of things to all kinds of people. A more specific goal would be: "When I get blood work done, I want all of my numbers to fall within the recommended range."

M – Measurable

In order to know that you have achieved your goal, it needs to be measurable in some way. For example, if you have a fitness goal, consider changing "I want to exercise more" to "I will be physically active an average of three to four days a week." Figure out what criteria success will be measured by for your goal.

A – Attainable

This one is pretty self-explanatory. Don't set an unrealistic, outlandish goal for yourself and expect to make it. You will only end up feeling like a failure. It is better to start small and build on your successes. Having several "wins" under your belt will propel you forward, maybe enabling you to achieve something you never could have done at the start.

R – Realistic

Making your goal realistic is similar to making it attainable but goes a step further. In addition to its being *possible* to achieve (attainable), you should also consider if you are at a place in your life where you are willing to do the work necessary to achieve it. No one else can reach your goals for you; it is something only you can do. Make sure that your goal is realistic for you at this point in time. If it's not, you can always shelve it and come back to it later on when you have more resources available to you.

T – Timely

Giving yourself a deadline will help increase your motivation and accountability to your goal. Come up with realistic but inspiring deadlines that propel you always forward. Consider mini-deadlines for the steps along the way to achieving your main goal. This will help keep you on track and ensure you meet your goal on time.

Your Future Timeline

Speaking of timeliness, let's do a little future-building exercise. Thinking about your future can help you clarify your goals and priorities. It can also free you from your day-to-day stresses and allow you to put the bulk of your attention into what really matters long-term in your life. Your answers in this exercise can involve food and wellness, but feel free to explore all the areas of your life.

Start by grabbing a piece of paper (maybe you've started working in a journal at this point!). Title it something like "Future Timeline." Next, write down all of the things that you would like to get done by the following deadlines:

- By the end of the day tomorrow
- This week
- This month
- This year
- Five years from now (What year will it be? How old will you be? What all do you want to have accomplished?)
- Ten years from now (What year will it be? How old will you be? What all do you want to have accomplished?)
- Twenty years from now (What year will it be? How old will you be? What all do you want to have accomplished?)

Really put some time into this. Once you have your Future Timeline, you can begin laying out your roadmap for achieving these goals.

Sub-Goals

Some of your goals might be big enough to consider making sub-goals. These smaller goals will guide you towards meeting a larger, related goal. Let's say you have the goal of being physically active three to four days per week on average. Well, if you are currently a couch potato, it's going to be pretty hard to jump right into an exercise program that has you working out three to four days a week right off the bat. This would be an instance where sub-goals would be helpful. Some potential sub-goals in this situation could be:

- Join a gym
- Explore various forms of movement (walking, yoga, dance, swimming, strength training, etc.) to see what appeals to you.
- Explore various formats for exercise (individual, partner, group exercise classes) to see what suits your personality best
- Start becoming more active in your day-to-day life (park farther out in the parking lot, take the stairs, etc.)
- Start with one to two days of activity, then build up to two to three, then three to four

This kind of method will have you making big changes slowly, and the change will be less burdensome and may even happen right under your nose! Many clients who work with me look back after six months and cannot believe how far they've come! They almost have forgotten their old ways! Sub-goals are a crucial part of this equation. Plus, they tend to result in lasting change because it has been so gradual, as opposed to all those January gym-goers that fall off the wagon come March.

Bumps in the Road

Inevitably, you will encounter obstacles to meeting your goals. Life is imperfect, and you cannot anticipate setbacks that may be lurking around the corner. That being said, there are potential obstacles that you may be able to foresee. It is helpful to think through these before they come up and have a strategy in place to overcome them. Think of it as a well-developed game plan. You have to read the defense, know your weaknesses, and come up with ideas on how to score nonetheless.

Anticipating potential obstacles is helpful with all of our goals—both short and long term—but, for the purposes of this exercise, let's look specifically at your goal(s) for one year from now. In your journal or on your piece of paper, write out each of your one-year goals. Next, begin brainstorming all the potential hurdles you may encounter in your journey to reach these goals and write them down. Here are some questions to get you thinking:

- What about this goal would be a challenge to anyone?
- What about my personality may make this more challenging?
- What about my situation at home, at work, and in my social life may present problems?
- What resources do I currently lack that are needed to achieve this goal?
- Do I have the support I need to reach my goal?

This exercise may feel a little "Debbie Downer," but worry not! We are about to put a positive spin on it.

You just spent some time thinking about how you may get tripped up, and now we are going to develop strategies to avoid these potential issues. For instance, let's say you have the goal of learning how to cook more nutritious food. An obstacle you may have come up with was that your family will likely resist being served different meals, especially if they know that they are "healthy." Great. This is not a deal-breaker, just a little obstacle that you can anticipate and come up with ways to overcome. Some ideas to remedy the situation could be:

- Tell your family that you are going to be trying some new recipes and can't wait to get their feedback. This makes them feel valued and involved in the process.
- Cook some of their old favorites, subbing in more

healthful ingredients.
- Give them ways to customize their dishes according to their preferences. Offer a variety of sauces, toppings, seasonings, etc.
- Get them cooking with you! Having them help to prepare a meal gives them ownership over it and will make them more likely to eat and enjoy it.

Do this for each of your goals, especially your goals for up to one year from now. That way, when issues arise—and they will—you won't sweat them because you will already have a plan in place.

Action Plan

Now that you have your goals, sub-goals, potential obstacles, and strategies to overcome those obstacles, you need to make your action plan. Your action plan is similar to the Future Timeline you completed, but focus on one goal at a time. Include a deadline for that goal and any sub-goals and their deadlines, as well. It may be helpful to schedule a time to specifically work on each goal. Also, make sure to include a space for your potential obstacles as well as your strategies to overcome them. This will function as the "Troubleshooting" section of your action plan.

The Benefits

Now is the time to let yourself really go there. Begin to imagine yourself achieving all of your goals. How would your life improve? Next to each goal, list out the benefits that would come from reaching it. Continuing with the above example of cooking healthier meals, some potential benefits could be:

- Weight loss
- Better blood work results
- Improved self-esteem

- Improvement in eating habits of spouse and children
- Increased energy and vitality

Do this for each of your goals and begin to see how life could be better. Hopefully you are feeling extra inspired. Don't you *really* want to achieve them now?

Get Outside Support

A crucial part of your success will be the support you have around you. Your spouse, parents, children, and friends can have a huge impact on your well-being and ability to achieve the goals you have for yourself. Hopefully your friends and family are in tune with your needs and fully support you. They can be excellent resources when you need to vent, bounce an idea around, or seek encouragement. They can even help you with meal planning, grocery shopping, and cooking. And once you are cooking delicious and nutritious meals, it probably won't take much convincing to get them to eat with you, either.

It will be helpful to sit them down and explain to them why you want to make a change in your life. Consider showing them some of the writing exercises you've done in your journal such as your Why Letter, Future Timeline, and the Benefits of reaching your goals. Giving them a glimpse into what motivates you deep down will help them understand your choices. They will probably be even more supportive and understanding than they otherwise would have been because they know what it means to you.

Maybe your loved ones need to make a change too and will be inspired by your journey. If you suspect this to be the case, then you can ask them if they would like to join you in trying to make these changes for themselves. If you are surrounded by others who are moving towards similar goals, it can be very motivating and provide additional accountability. Couples, in particular, tend to be more successful when both partners are committed to the process, as opposed to when only one is trying to make a change. Get your tribe on your side.

It is also definitely possible that the people in your life will not be supportive. If this is the case, don't let it get you down. Watching another person make lifestyle changes can be threatening to people, because they become more aware of the areas that could use improvement in their own lives. Even if you think they could benefit from change, back off if they seem reluctant. They have to be ready for it to work, and you don't want them to resent you for being too pushy.

If your friends and family aren't on board with what you are doing, you may have less support initially, but think about it as an opportunity to lead by example. When people see the positive changes happening in your life, they will likely be inspired themselves. At a minimum, they will see that what you are doing is having a positive change on your life and will have a hard time arguing against that. Be a light for those around you.

Visualize Your Success

Visualization is the act of imagining something that is not actually happening in front of you. People use this technique for all kinds of reasons, such as stress management and inducing sleep, but it can also be very helpful for reaching your wellness and food goals.

You've probably already used visualization, even if it wasn't on purpose. When you considered the benefits of reaching your goals, you probably envisioned yourself in the future, having met them. You imagined how you would look, feel, and behave. That's visualization!

While visualization can be a tool for meeting your goals,

many people can inadvertently sabotage themselves using visualization. Have you ever been nervous about a future event, and spent a lot of time leading up to it imagining the worst-case scenario? Did the event go well for you? Probably not, or at least, it didn't go as well as it could have.

This goes back to your beliefs. What we believe, we create. Visualization helps you create the belief that you not only *can* achieve your goals, but it helps you *believe* that you *will* achieve your goals. So, how do you do it?

First, set up a conducive environment to visualization. A quiet, dimly lit room with minimal distractions works well. Next, get comfortable. Dress comfortably, and either sit or lie down on a cozy chair, couch, or yoga mat. Take a few deep breaths, and close your eyes.

Begin by setting up a mental image of yourself achieving your goal. What does that look like for you? Notice how you feel. What do you see? What do you hear from yourself and those around you? Try to imagine the scene through all of your senses. Really immerse yourself in it.

You can even take on more specific scenes. One technique is to use visualization to overcome any obstacles before you encounter them. Pull out your Obstacles List and the strategies you came up with for conquering them. Visualize each scenario playing out and you successfully using each of the strategies you came up with.

Example Visualization

Maybe you have the goal of not overeating past the point when you are full, and you know that social settings where food is out all night long can be a stumbling block for you. Your strategy could be to eat ahead of time so that you aren't overly hungry, and then allow yourself one plateful of foods that are the most appealing to you at the party. You then will spend the rest of the event engaged in conversation away from the food table.

So, instead of just writing out this obstacle and strategy, *visualize* it. Imagine yourself preparing for an upcoming party. What will you wear? How do you do your hair and makeup? Imagine having a small meal or snack before you head out the door. What do you eat? How does that taste? Smile, knowing that before you even enter the party, you've done something to set yourself up for success.

You arrive at the party. Where is it? Who else is there? What kind of sounds do you hear? Conversation? Laughter? Music? Who greets you, and what do they say? Who are you most excited to spend time with at the party? Go find that person and strike up a conversation. Spend time saying hello and chatting with the other attendees.

Next, think about the smells—oh, the smells! Notice what foods are being offered. Are they appetizing? What colors do you see? What textures? Maybe the food looks amazing, or maybe it looks just fair. Think about that for a second. Does the food even look good? If it does, great, but if not, consider whether you really want any of it at all. You did eat ahead of time—remember?

If some of it looks really good, allow yourself one plateful. What do you put on that plate? How much of each item? Then, picture yourself walking away from the food table to eat and continue visiting with everyone at the party. Enjoy every bite and notice how everything tastes. Does each item taste as good as you expected it to? If it is delicious, really savor everything about it. Enjoy the texture, aroma, and how it lights up your taste buds as you roll it around in your mouth. If it doesn't taste that good, consider stopping after one bite. Let the conversation, not the food, be your focus for the night.

Imagine the end of the party and your drive home. What did you enjoy most about the party? Who did you have good conversations with? What foods did you enjoy eating? How do you feel having overcome that obstacle? How does this propel you further towards accomplishing your goals?

Do this kind of visualization with all of your goals and perceived obstacles whenever something comes up that brings on stress or makes you doubt your resolve. See yourself being successful, and it is more likely to happen. Practice visualization because the more you do it, the better you will be and the more it will impact you in a positive way.

Consider some alternative "visualization" techniques. For example, try writing out your visualization, just as if you were imagining it, but put it into words. Use the present tense as if it is really happening to you, right now. Be as descriptive as possible.

Another idea is to make a Dream Board. You can cut out pictures, words, recipes, etc., from magazines and other print materials and paste those cutouts on a poster board to create an artifact of your visualization. You can even create a virtual board on Pinterest that can serve the same purpose. Having something concrete that you can revisit to inspire yourself can be very helpful. You can always tweak it along the way if your goals evolve.

Consider a Reward

Lastly, consider a reward for meeting your goals. If you are trying to overcome some unhealthy eating habits, I wouldn't recommend using food as a reward—that may have gotten you into this problem in the first place! Instead, think about alternatives. Maybe you want to get your nails done or buy yourself that purse you've been eyeing for some time now. Your reward could also be something as extravagant as a vacation or as simple as a bubble bath. Make a promise to yourself that when you meet your goal, you will give yourself a reward and be specific about what that reward will be.

15. BECOME INTENTIONAL

In the previous chapter, we discussed goal-setting, which is an important skill in life. Goals help to motivate us and to give us an idea of where we are going, but they can be too big-picture and future-focused to help us grow in the present moment. For that, we need intentions.

Intentions, unlike goals, are present-oriented. They are helpful to redirect and center you on what you have identified to be most important. They can help align you with your values and can assist you when outside forces threaten to throw you off course. When stressful or emotional situations arise, it can be hard to continue pursuing your goals in those moments. Intentions bring you back, even in the midst of the storm.

Even when you act in a way that is not aligned with your goals, your intentions function as the quiet reminders, allowing you to forgive yourself but go back to behaving in a way that is in concert with your beliefs. While goals are focused on external results, intentions focus on internal guidance. In addition, success in goal-setting has everything to do with the end result—did you meet your goal? With intention-setting, success has more to do with how well your daily choices match up with your values. Did you live your beliefs? Even if you do something that is out of balance with your intentions, you can always come back to them. Intentions are not as black and white as goals are.

Spiritual practices utilize various forms of intention setting to help guide believers. Christians memorize Bible verses to summon at will when a particular situation applies. Hindus and Buddhists use mantras, which are sacred words or phrases, to guide their spiritual practices.

Intentions can be very similar to your goals, but they tend to have more to do with ongoing choices and behaviors, as opposed to one end result. For instance, you may have the goal of getting your blood work numbers normalized—that is one end result. Did you or didn't you?

Intentions, on the other hand, give opportunities every day to choose to act on them. They tend to be aligned with your goals, and may even function like sub-goals or stepping stones towards larger goals for your future. Some examples of possible intentions are:

- I intend to spread love and happiness in my interactions with others.
- I intend to lead by example.
- I intend to love my food.
- I intend to release myself from guilt.
- I intend to forgive others and myself.
- I intend to choose more colorful foods.
- I intend to learn more about cooking.

Do you see the difference? Learning how to develop and call upon these intentions can be very influential in your day-to-day life. The more you practice intention-setting, the better you will become at actually living your values and beliefs.

How to Set an Intention

First, you need to come up with an intention. It is helpful if your intention is focused on the present, something that you can immediately start applying to your life. Maybe your goals could give you ideas for related intentions, or maybe they are unrelated. Consider spending some time in prayer or quiet meditation, quieting your mind a bit to come up with your Intention. Think about your beliefs and values. Read your Why List/Letter. All of these things will help to give you ideas about what your Intention should be.

Length is also important. You don't want something that is long and tedious because, ultimately, it would be nice if you could memorize your Intention. Simplicity is key—it is much easier to live your Intention if it is simple.

Focus on just one intention at first. If you set more than one, you may have a hard time living it out fully at first. Once you have practiced using intentions to guide your life, you can consider setting more than one at a time. For now, start with one.

Once you have come up with your Intention, write it down on a small notecard and put it in your pocket, purse, briefcase—wherever you will have it with you throughout the day. Whenever you think about it, pull out this Intention Notecard and read it. Close your eyes a moment, focusing on the words of your Intention, and bring yourself back. Think about how you can apply it to that specific moment in front of you.

It is likely that you will occasionally catch yourself acting in a way that is out of alignment with your Intention. We are imperfect. Stress happens, old habits arise, and other people tick us off—"best-laid plans often go awry," as they say. The key is to notice the discrepancy between your current behavior and your Intention and redirect yourself. Repeat your Intention and modify your behavior. Then forgive yourself and move forward.

Grounding Yourself in Your Intention

Using your Intention Notecard is a great start, but to best immerse yourself in your Intention, you may consider going a step further. As mentioned above, using prayer or meditation can be helpful in coming up with your Intention. Prayer and meditation can also be beneficial in really grounding yourself in it. It is one thing to have some words written out in your pocket and another to spend some quiet time, free of distractions, really pondering your Intention and letting it sink in.

Think about devoting even just five minutes each morning to quietly contemplating your Intention. Repeat it over and over to yourself. Focus specifically on each word in your Intention and think about what the words mean to you. Remember ways in which you have lived out your Intention in the past. Look at your plans for the day ahead and imagine ways in which you may be able to make choices that are in line with your Intention. Examine the potential benefits of acting from your Intention today. Think about how others may be positively affected by your actions today as well.

You can also use time before meals to set your Intention, especially if your Intention has something to do with food or eating. Take a moment to pause and reflect. Think about why you set that Intention in the first place and how you will let it guide your eating and the rest of your meal experience. Then, enjoy the food in front of you and the company you are sharing it with!

Check In With Yourself

Not everything is rainbows and roses, and there are going to be situations that arise that test your intentions. In fact, especially at the beginning you may feel like you are taking one step forward and two steps back. That is okay! Be patient and forgiving with yourself. We are *all* works in progress. Decide to let it go and look ahead. Pull out your Intention Notecard, read back over your journal, meditate, take a walk—whatever you need to do to clear your head, center yourself, and reclaim the moment.

You may come to a point where you are feeling awfully comfortable—or maybe even bored—with your Intention. It is possible that you've mastered it. That's great! It's likely that you won't feel very inspired anymore using the same one, so determine a new Intention and apply the same steps above to start living it out.

It is also possible that your goals or values have changed, and your intention needs some modifying to better suit your needs. That's great, too. Make the process work for you, so you are constantly working towards a better version of the "you" that you want to be.

Moving Forward

As we wrap up Part Two, check in with yourself. Are you ready to incorporate the action steps needed to heal your relationship with food or do you need to spend some more time working on the mental part? Be really honest with yourself. It is okay to continue working and reworking on the steps in Part Two before moving on to Part Three. In fact, that would be preferred if you aren't quite ready to start incorporating the eating and food changes. If you move on too quickly without having gone through the necessary internal shifts, you will likely relapse into your old ways of thinking and behaving with food. Do not worry. Part Three will be waiting for you whenever you are ready.

If, on the other hand, you are feeling the internal shifts happening and you are ready to incorporate the physical, action-oriented strategies, go ahead and read on.

PART THREE:
LESS TALK, MORE ACTION

LINDSAY REINHOLT

16. PUTTING IT INTO PRACTICE

In the previous section, the focus was on the internal shifts that are necessary to make change that *lasts*. You were encouraged to dig deep to discover your "why" for this journey, the real motivation for your thirst for change. You examined and challenged the beliefs that you had coming into this process and developed more positive beliefs based on *truth*. In addition, you learned to appreciate the good and unique things about your body's appearance and function, and not to dwell on the things that you wish were different. Next, you took a hard look at the messages that surround you and how they can have a positive or negative effect on your self-esteem and goals for your life. This prompted you to be more discerning with these influences and maybe consider getting rid of some of the ones that aren't in line with helping you reaching your goals. You were also encouraged to say "good-bye" to guilt surrounding your food choices and embrace each bump in the road as a learning opportunity rather than a failure. Educating yourself on the food system, nutrition, and other eating and health topics was also discussed as a further means of motivation and giving purpose to the changes you are making. Lastly, you set goals for yourself to create a path to success and intentions to help you live more aligned with your values.

Whew! That was a lot of work—good work, necessary work, work that will yield lasting results. Don't you feel better already? You should. In many ways, the internal work is the hardest, and, once it's complete, the next part comes fairly naturally. You will still come up against obstacles, but if you stay rooted in what you worked on in Part Two, you will make progress and ultimately find success.

In Part Three, you will begin to take action and make changes to your eating patterns. You will likely be changing some habits that are pretty deeply ingrained, which won't always be comfortable, but I encourage you to be open to the process. Tweak these suggestions to make them work for you and your personality and situation, but always come back to your Why, your Goals, and your Intentions.

17. BECOME AN OBSERVER OF YOURSELF

Your first task is simply to become an observer of you. Many of our eating habits and food choices are subconscious— we don't really think much about them. They are habits that we have had for years, often developing during childhood. When you take a step back, though, and really start to notice and think about the choices you make, you can begin to rethink and redefine them. You may even realize that they aren't as healthy or body-honoring as you would like.

The Food Diary

You will begin by starting a food diary. *Oh no, she's going to make me track everything I eat,* you are probably thinking. Yep, I sure am. The thing is, this food diary is not meant to serve as your Calorie Police, making sure you stop at any certain point. It is purely to keep track of what you are eating and when, for observational purposes only. I am not asking you to change anything right now.

Write down all of your meals, snacks, and nibbles throughout the day, noting the time when you eat each one. Do this for a few days or a couple weeks, whatever works for you, until you feel like you have a good sampling of your eating habits.

Once you've collected this information, look over your diary and make note of the following things:

- Are there any particular foods you eat regularly, like every day?
- Is there any pattern to your eating? Do you eat more or less during certain parts of the day?
- Which foods do you love? Which foods do you not like that much? Why do you think you eat certain foods that you don't love?
- How do external forces affect your eating choices? Were there certain social events, stressful situations, or outside pressures that encouraged you to eat in a way you wouldn't have otherwise?

As you think about these questions with regard to your food diary, also consider how your eating choices relate to your Why, your Goals, and your Intentions. Do you see a need for changes anywhere? Identify the moments where your food choices did not line up with your Why, Goals, and Intentions.

Hunger

Now it is time to add the next step. Previously, you have simply recorded your food choices and the times at which you ate. Now, you are going to record your hunger. Again, this is simply observational. You are still allowed to eat even if you are not particularly hungry.

Let's address a little bit about hunger before you begin. Hunger can be a tricky thing because it is often a subtle sensation, one to which many people are not attuned. If you've spent many years eating too much or eating when you were not hungry, you may have a difficult time recognizing hunger in the first place. In order to eat mindfully and in a way that nourishes and loves your body, you will need to understand your hunger and use it to guide your eating choices *most* of the time.

So, what is hunger? Hunger is simply your body telling you that it needs more fuel. Fuel comes in the form of calories. Calories are energy and necessary for your survival—they are not evil and to be avoided at all costs. If you learn to listen to your body and eat mindfully, you will naturally eat the right amount of calories for your unique body and your unique lifestyle. No counting necessary! Whew!

The key is to eat in a way that is hunger-driven. There is a particular window of opportunity where you are neither satisfied nor starving, and that is the perfect time to grab a bite. I call this The Golden Hour. If you eat during The Golden Hour, you are more likely to eat in a way that is healthy and controlled. That is ideal. On the other hand, if you get too hungry, you will enter The Danger Zone, where you will be more likely to eat too much food and choose foods that you wouldn't otherwise choose—like cookies, pizza, and chips. When you get into The Danger Zone, all your brain can think about is, "MUST EAT NOW!" Not good if you are trying to eat healthfully.

Hunger is a gradual thing. It starts very subtly—usually with just an inkling that food sounds desirable. You may even question whether the sensations you are feeling are hunger at all. And they may not be! You may just be thirsty or bored. Have a glass of water and find something productive or fun to do, and revisit the question of food in twenty minutes or so. If you are still feeling unsatisfied or the sensations have intensified, maybe you really are hungry!

The feelings we often associate with hunger—stomach pangs, churning, and shakiness—are actually products of being overly hungry. If you start feeling those, you've entered The Danger Zone. You can certainly still make good eating choices in The Danger Zone, but it is much more difficult because your body is now experiencing stress, which makes it quite hard to make good decisions. The best tip is to have healthy, quick foods prepared and ready to go so that you can meet your hunger needs right away and not grab a less-healthy alternative instead.

So, now that you know what hunger is and how to identify it, you should begin recording it in your food diary each time you eat. The best way to do this is to use a Hunger Scale.

The Hunger Scale

There are many hunger scales out there, and they all serve basically the same purpose—to help people identify how hungry they are at any given moment. Many times these scales are just too big, making it overly difficult to use them effectively. I think a simple, five-point scale is best. Here's the one I use with my clients:

1 – Stuffed, uncomfortable, and food no longer sounds good

2 – Full but comfortable, satisfied

3 – Neither full nor hungry, neutral

4 – Hungry, there's a slight emptiness to the stomach, food is desirable, subtle hunger sensations in the mouth and stomach; The Golden Hour

5 – Overly hungry, starving, ravenous, stomach pangs, shakiness, and other unpleasant sensations; The Danger Zone

So, there you have it. Simple enough, right? Ideally, you should aim to eat when at around a 4. That is the optimal time when you are both hungry enough to eat, but also not so far gone that you'll plow your way through a box of Ho Hos.

Begin recording your meals and snacks, each time putting a

number from the Hunger Scale that corresponds to your level of hunger at the time of eating. Again, this is not to say you have to be at a 4 or 5 every time you eat (though a 4 is preferable!). You can still eat even if you are not hungry. No one is telling you that you can't, but be mindful. Be aware. The whole purpose of using your food diary is to learn more about your own habits to better inform your future decisions. You are not using it to become a perfectionist or feel like a failure every time you eat at a number other than a 4, but through recording your hunger and food choices you should become more aware of the results of eating at different levels of hunger.

Using the Hunger Scale with Your Food Diary to Redirect your Eating Cues

Now that you are including hunger in your observations, take a look at your diary and note:

- At which number do I most often eat?
- Is there a time of day when I tend to eat before reaching a 4?
- What reasons might I have for eating when I am not hungry?
- Do I ever reach a 5? Why? When does this most often occur? How can I avoid it?
- What do my food choices look like at each number on the scale? Do I tend to eat certain kinds of foods at a 3, 4, or 5?

If this has been a difficult exercise, that is okay! Eating for non-hunger reasons is probably one of the leading contributors to your less-than-stellar relationship with food, and it can be a painful wake-up call when you shine a light on it. It also takes time to undo some of those automatic habits you have about when and what to eat.

Now that you have taken a good look at your initial habits,

and analyzed them and looked for patterns, it is time to think about some of the eating cues you need to ditch. For instance, did your food diary inform you that you tend to have a 9:00 p.m. snack every evening, regardless of whether or not you are hungry? Maybe for you it is a 3:00 p.m. snack that you use as a reward for making it through most of your day at work. These timed snacks tend to be something very automatic and not hunger-driven. For me, it was the 9:00 p.m. snack. I would literally wait until 9:00 p.m. rolled around, exactly, and then it was time for a treat—something sweet and usually not very nutritious. It's a hard habit to break, but here are some ideas to play with:

- Replace your snack with another activity that you can look forward to such as a walk, a game, writing in a journal, reading a book, doing your nails, etc.
- Drink tea instead of having a snack.
- Allow yourself a small portion of something that you love, like a piece of dark chocolate. Whatever you choose, make sure to portion it out so that you are having a small amount that still meets your needs.

Of course, if you are genuinely hungry, eat something, but don't wait until your designated time to eat if you get hungry before that. Shoot for a 4, remember! Check in with yourself and think about what your body really needs. Think about giving it the fuel it needs to continue functioning at its best.

Another problem people come up against is getting way too hungry between meals. If your goal is to eat at a 4 most of the time, you may need to consider eating more frequently than you are used to doing. Everybody is different and has a different metabolism. Again, if you look at it through the car-and-gas metaphor, some cars burn through fuel more quickly than others do. Maybe you get great mileage, maybe you are a "gas-guzzler," or maybe you fall somewhere between. The point is, for many people, eating breakfast at 7:00 a.m., lunch at noon, and dinner at

6:00 p.m., is not enough. So, experiment with it! Prepare yourself a healthy morning snack and a healthy afternoon snack. Try eating more frequent, smaller meals per day. Sometimes, I like to split a meal in half, eating part of it when I first start getting hungry and saving the rest for about an hour later when I get hungry again. Find what works for you and tweak it as you go.

Maybe your problem isn't that you associate certain *times of day* with eating; maybe your problem is that you associate certain *activities* with eating. For many, watching TV goes hand-in-hand with having something to munch on. Maybe the second you walk in the door from work, you gravitate toward the kitchen. Whatever it is for you, rethink what you *actually* need in that moment. Maybe it isn't food after all. If you are watching TV, you are probably just bored and looking for an escape. Consider an alternative activity, one that involves other people even, that can captivate you. Play a game, get into a creative project, do something for someone else. Try to distract yourself from the desire to eat if you aren't actually hungry.

Remember, these are habits, and, as such, they are difficult to break. It will likely feel quite uncomfortable at first, and you will probably have some setbacks along the way. Give yourself grace to make mistakes, and move on. The more you rethink your habits and eat for hunger as opposed to other reasons, the more you will honor your Why, Goals, and Intentions, and the easier it will get.

Recognizing Fullness

We've spent a lot of time discussing when to *start* eating, but now we need to think about when to *stop*. Hunger and fullness are inextricably intertwined. In an ideal world, you eat when you start feeling hungry, and you stop eating when you first start feeling satisfied. "Fullness" is a difficult feeling to understand, especially if you have spent years eating to the point of feeling stuffed and uncomfortable. Maybe your cue to stop eating shouldn't be, "I feel full," but rather, "I feel satisfied."

Like hunger, fullness is a spectrum, and the sensation is gradual. There is a difference between feeling satisfied and feeling stuffed. The goal is satisfaction, not having to unbuckle your top button and go lie down for a few minutes after you finish.

It is commonly understood that it takes your brain about twenty minutes to register fullness. As you eat and then start to digest that food, certain events initiate the creation of hormones in your GI tract that get sent to the brain to tell you to stop eating. The problem, though, is that if you eat too quickly, your brain doesn't have enough time to receive the signal. Cue the bloat and regret.

Focus on slowing down during your meal. Enjoy the experience and don't rush through it just to move on to the next activity. Chew your food slowly. Go through each component of your meal as if you were a food critic. Thoughtfully consider each bite. What do you like? What don't you like? What flavors do you notice? Be discerning.

Another important thing to realize is this: You are NOT going to starve. This is not your last meal, so don't eat like it is. There is almost always food available to you, and you have permission to eat whenever you need to. It's a strange phenomenon, but people often eat like a famine could be around the corner at any moment. *I don't want to get hungry later, so I better finish my plate*, you may think as you shovel those last few bites down. In reality, though, that food won't serve its intended purpose. Your body can't use all those calories at once, so off it will go, to your fat stores. And no matter how much you eat in one sitting, you will still get hungry later.

You also have to disassociate having a clean plate from being done. Were you a member of the Clean Plate Club growing up? Did your well-meaning parents encourage you to consume every morsel before you were allowed to leave the table? Look, the truth is, their parents probably did the same thing. Those generations lived during a time where food scarcity was a real problem and waste was a non-option. Fortunately for you, that is probably not the case. Food is available at all hours of the day or night, 365 days a year, and for relatively inexpensive prices. I'm not encouraging throwing tons of good food away, but remember this: Your body can only use a certain amount of fuel at any given time. The rest goes straight to your belly, buns, and hips. Maybe you didn't "waste" it by throwing it in the trash, but it certainly is "wasted" calories that will be converted to excess fat, and you will now have to work extra hard to get rid of them.

I was definitely a member of the Clean Plate Club growing up, and it is still a challenge for me to leave food on my plate. I have found that what works best for me is to start with smaller portions, actually *less* than I think I will want to eat. The food will still be there if I want more when I have finished. Sometimes I go back for more, but oftentimes I don't, finding the smaller portion was enough to satisfy me when all is said and done.

Another thing I have learned is the art of leftovers. Leftovers really are worth embracing. They make preparing lunch the next day a breeze, cut waste, reduce expenses, and discourage overeating. Plus, some foods even get better after a day or two in the fridge. (Pasta and soup are two of my favorites because of this!) One thing I do that I also recommend to my clients is to invest in some single-portion containers. As you are serving up your meal, portion out any extras into these as well. That way, you have already prepped your leftovers, they can cool for a bit before you put them in the refrigerator, and you will be less inclined to go back for more unless you are really still hungry. You'll thank yourself the next morning too when you already have a single serving of stir-fry packed up and ready to go for lunch that day.

Restaurants are notorious for super-size portions, and these can really expand your waistline, especially if dining out is a regular thing for you. Help yourself out and ask for a box right off the bat, putting away half of your meal before you even dive in. I don't remember the last time I ate out at a restaurant and didn't bring home enough leftovers from *one* meal to count as a whole additional meal the next day. Remember, this meal isn't your last. You can always eat more if you get hungry when you get home.

Remember to utilize your Food Diary and the Hunger Scale in helping you observe your behaviors and food choices. Learn from those choices and think about what you may want to change. Try to incorporate some of the tips I've included here to help you with eating when you are hungry, and avoiding eating otherwise.

18. FIND ACCOUNTABILITY

Accountability is a crucial component to success. This process isn't always going to be fun or easy. There will be tough times when you need some outside support to push you through. These are when having someone who can hold you accountable will be helpful.

Who to Choose

Ideally, a spouse, family member, or roommate could be your accountability partner. This option is great because this person usually lives with you and is more aware of your food choices. They can celebrate your successes and pull you back up when you stumble. They can also call you out if you lose sight of your Goals and Intentions and need some gentle correction.

In some situations, the person or people you live with may not be the best choice for accountability. They may be fearful of change in you as it may highlight some of their own issues with food. Jealousy could also be an issue if they see positive improvements in you and resent you for them. They may also be too harsh and judgmental to offer the gentle correction you need. If one of these is the case, then look for a close friend with values that line up with your goals. Another wonderful option is to begin working with a health professional that specializes in lifestyle change, such as a health coach.

Only you can know who in your life will offer the best support, but whomever you choose, make sure that they fully understand your goals. Make sure they support a non-judgmental approach that is flexible and slow-paced. Better yet, have them read this book and your journal, which will help them to understand exactly how you are working toward your goals and the steps you are taking to get there. Maybe even encourage someone in your life to consider taking this journey with you so that you could support each other as accountability partners.

How to Establish an Accountability Relationship

Obviously, the first step is to approach the person and ask them to support you in this way. If they are also on their own health journey, offer to do the same thing for them.

Next, get specific about what you will need from them. This looks different for everyone. Maybe you want to swap healthy recipes. Maybe you want them specifically to call you out if you seem to be eating for non-hunger reasons. Maybe you would like a daily or weekly phone call where you can simply share what is working and what is not and have a sounding board for any issues that come up. Really get clear about what support looks like to you, and share that with them to see if they would be willing and are able to do it.

After you confirm that they are in, open up. You need to share what got you to this point and how you are looking to approach this journey. The best way to do this is to go through your journal with them, specifically sharing your Why, your Goals, and your Intention. Help them take a look inside your headspace; invite them in. Doing this will not only help them to feel more informed on how best to help you but also will make them feel more invested in your success.

Make sure that they are 100-percent committed to helping you through this time. This is why working with a health coach can be so beneficial. Having someone independent from your personal and professional lives, whose sole purpose is to help you meet your health goals, can be very powerful. See the end of this book for more information on health coaches and how to get this kind of support.

Avoid the Naysayers and Food Pushers

As mentioned above, it is possible, maybe even likely, that not everyone in your life will be thrilled with your desire for change. Hearing about others' quest for better health can often bring up insecurities in people, especially if they perceive you as already healthier, thinner, or more attractive than they are. This can happen very easily, regardless of how much you share with them about your changes. You may have done nothing wrong, but they resent you nonetheless.

That being said, you should be aware of this possibility and be understanding of the people around you. We all have our own story and our own baggage, and many people simply aren't ready to make drastic changes in their lives. You are ready, and that is FABULOUS, but it doesn't mean you need to go around flaunting it for the world to see. Be honest and matter-of-fact with people if the situation warrants it; otherwise, "you do you," as they say, and don't pry into the business of others.

As a defense mechanism, some of these people may attempt to sabotage your success, whether they are aware of it or not. They may offer you more food than you want, talk negatively about healthy living, or share stories about people they know who failed trying to change their eating habits. These are the voices that you must avoid at all costs. They are toxic to your success.

If this is the case for you, give yourself permission to take a break from these relationships or at least to take a step back and minimize the time you spend together. As you become more solid in your new choices and routines, you will probably be able to resume activity with these people once again without its causing setbacks or harming your well-being.

It may also be a good opportunity to take a hard look at some of these relationships and see if they are worth holding onto in the long term. People come and go in our lives, and that is *okay*. It is okay to have friendships that last only seasons and to have others that last a lifetime. It is a healthy thing to reassess any relationship that brings you down more often than it brings you up and, potentially, to consider ending those relationships. Seek out other people that are more like-minded; better yet, find friends who inspire you to be better than you already are.

19. THE CAUSES OF CRAVINGS

Nobody can give you wiser advice than yourself.

--Cicero

Cravings. We all have them. For the dieter, cravings are the worst nightmare. They threaten to unravel all of their good work and send them down the rabbit hole of overeating and choosing foods that don't support their goals.

When we get cravings, they are usually for foods like chocolate, pizza, and chips, not asparagus. Many people describe themselves as "sweet" people or "salty" people. "Sweet" people crave sweet foods like cookies and candy, and "salty" people crave french fries, chips, and other savory morsels. It is actually possible, although not as common, to crave nutritious foods. In my early twenties, when I was backpacking through Europe, I remember getting cravings for raw produce, like salads and fruit, since most of my meals were made up of cooked fare or easy items from the market, like cheese, cured meats, and olives.

What are Cravings and What Causes Them?

Cravings are simply a message from your body telling you that something is out of balance. Your body wants to maintain

109

homeostasis, and cravings are a way that it does this. Cravings can come about as a result of a physical trigger or an emotional trigger.

Physical Triggers

Physical triggers include nutrient deficiencies, low blood sugar, dehydration, lack of sleep, hormones, the current season of the year, addiction, survival instincts, and restriction.

Nutrient Deficiencies

Despite our fairly large intake of calories, many people are actually deficient in some nutrients. We eat a lot of stuff, but oftentimes not enough of the *essential* stuff that helps our bodies to function optimally. Our bodies respond through cravings for foods that have those nutrients. For instance, did you know that cravings for salty food could indicate a lack of iodine in the body and chocolate cravings are often a sign of a magnesium deficiency? Your body really is so smart!

Low Blood Sugar

Blood sugar regulation is another issue that can feed into cravings. If your blood sugar drops too low, you are more likely to have cravings. Sugar cravings can actually be the body's request for more protein, which will help to stabilize the blood sugar, leading to fewer surges and drops and making you feel satisfied for longer with fewer cravings. You may also consider eating more regularly. As discussed in the section on The Hunger Scale in Chapter 17, getting overly hungry can send you down a dark road where you succumb to each craving that comes along. Work to balance your blood sugar.

Dehydration

Another potential cause of your cravings is dehydration.

Your body needs a lot of water throughout the day to function properly. Most people do not drink enough. Dehydration can manifest itself as mild hunger and cravings. Grab a glass of water and see if that squelches your craving first.

Lack of Sleep

Have you ever had a particularly rough day of cravings after a rough night of sleep? A lack of sleep has been shown to increase cravings for carbs and sweets the following day, so consider getting some more shut-eye to ward off your cravings. Many people have a hard time prioritizing sleep and try to justify a late bed time. In reality, though, you are fighting your internal clock, which can cause all kinds of problems for you. A few of these potential issues include weakened immune system, dampened cognitive processing, increased chance of all kinds of health issues like heart disease and diabetes, lowered sex drive, increased incidence of depression and anxiety, greater likelihood of weight gain, and more. It may not feel like you have enough hours in the day, but clocking some shut eye will certainly feel better during your waking hours and help your short- and long-term health significantly.

Hormonal Changes

Hormones can have a huge effect on cravings. Many women report having certain cravings at different times during their menstrual cycles or during menopause. It is difficult to combat these cravings, but you *should* work to become aware of them. Consider keeping track of them in your food diary so that you can be aware of when they are likely to hit and plan accordingly with healthier alternatives to the foods you normally crave.

Seasonality

Something most people don't think too much about is seasonality of food. Have you ever thought about why strawberries are so darn expensive in the winter and the shelves get stocked with squash and apples on sale in the fall? Seasonality, my friend!

Thanks to nature, different produce items are at peak for harvest at different times of the year. Citrus, root vegetables, and cabbage are best in the winter; artichokes and asparagus are springtime vegetables; berries, peaches, corn, green beans, and melons are examples of summer harvest plants; and fall is good for pears, apples, squash, and sweet potatoes.

It wasn't that long ago that people had to abide by nature when selecting the produce items that they ate. People ate what could be grown locally at different times of the year. If you lived in Minnesota, you probably didn't have access to tropical fruits such as pineapple and you only had berries during the summer.

We now live in a different era. Because of farms in warm-climate countries and the ability to treat produce to prevent early spoilage and ship it across the globe, we now have access to most produce throughout the year, regardless of seasonality.

Despite this, our bodies *prefer* to eat seasonally. I know I tend to crave warm, roasted root vegetables like sweet potatoes and Brussels sprouts (a member of the cabbage family) in the winter, and I prefer fresh, raw salads and crunchy cucumbers in the summer. Our bodies like to use foods to warm us when we are cold and cool us when we are hot. Root vegetables, which are grown in the soil, tend to have a warming, grounding effect on us, which is very comforting when it's frosty outside. Salads are full of water and energizing nutrients that cool us off and make us feel refreshed when we are hot.

Thinking beyond produce, in the winter, our bodies crave warm foods with higher fat contents. This is something that we've inherited from our ancestors. In order to survive the cold winter months when little food would be available, they needed to eat calorically dense foods full of fat. This mainly came in the form of animals that they would hunt and eat. Today, meats, casseroles, and stews all meet this need for the modern-day man.

Lastly, in the summer we look for lighter protein options, things like chicken and seafood. Paying attention to the seasonality of food when making your choices will help ward off cravings that your body sends to bring balance into this area.

Addiction

Another reason for cravings is slightly more sinister. Addiction can lead to cravings. *You can't be addicted to food*, you may be thinking. Or can you? Many foods cause very similar reactions to other substances that are widely recognized as addictive, like drugs and alcohol (which actually falls into the category of food/drink.)

Did you know that sugar causes dopamine to be released into the brain? Dopamine is the neurotransmitter associated with pleasure, and it is the same thing that makes people addicted to heroin. Granted, much more dopamine is released with heroin, but too much sugar at one time can certainly trigger a series of events that can lead to a sugar addiction to a certain degree.

Similarly, it has been found that the digestion of casein (a dairy protein) produces casomorphins, which can have an opiate effect on the brain, causing you to want more and more. You really can become addicted to cheese! Furthermore, research has shown that some additives in processed foods can be addictive to certain people.

Survival Instincts

Up until a very recent time in history, human beings had to fight for food. Famine, migration of animals, natural disasters, and winter all affected the access we had to plants and animals. The people that survived were the ones who ate enough and were best able to store a lot of that food as fat. The best food for storage is fatty and calorically dense food. You don't have to eat as much of this kind of food to get plenty of calories. Thus, our DNA is preprogrammed to crave fatty and sugary foods that pack on the pounds—for survival, of course.

The problem is that now there are three McDonald's in a two-mile radius of your house, a grocery store five minutes down the road, and pizza a phone call away. We live in an environment with an overabundance of food, but our bodies still think that we are hunter-gatherers preparing for a long, cold winter. Add that to a dieting mentality, where you are constantly avoiding fatty or sugary foods, and your body will go into overdrive, blasting you with intense cravings that are nearly impossible to ignore. Your body wants you to *survive*, remember?

Restriction

The last physical trigger I would like to mention is restriction. As discussed at the beginning of this book in the chapter about dieting, restriction causes all kinds of problems. Besides slowing the metabolism, causing rebound binge-eating, and creating all kinds of emotional and mental issues surrounding food, it also can cause cravings. If you are on a strict diet with a giant list of "no-no" foods, you are more than likely going to start craving those exact foods in no time. Suddenly, all you can think about are ice cream and pizza. Truly, the most sure-fire way to get a craving is to tell yourself that you aren't allowed to eat that particular food. It is almost a guarantee at that point.

Emotional Triggers

Emotional triggers include stress, boredom, emotional repression, comfort or longing for home, and being unsatisfied in your personal or professional life.

Stress

Have you ever craved sugar when you are stressed or upset about something? Carbohydrates (i.e. sugar) boost the body's levels of serotonin, a neurotransmitter that is associated with happiness and wellbeing. Eating cake really does make you feel better—for a short time, anyway. The problem is, after the food is gone and your serotonin high has waned, the emotional trigger is still there. You didn't handle the actual cause of your stress.

Boredom

Using food as a distraction or entertainment is very common. If you don't have anything else to do, boredom can absolutely push you to snoop in the kitchen for a treat. This most often occurs during the afternoon and nighttime, and also commonly happens during transitions between activities.

Emotional Repression

When you have feelings that you don't express, they can manifest themselves as cravings. It is important to find healthy outlets for your emotions that don't involve food. You may find it helpful to talk to a close friend, relative, or therapist. Journaling, art, and physical activity can also be fantastic. Make sure that you feel heard and understood in your life by those around you; if you don't, then open up a dialogue to work through that.

Comfort or Longing for Home

We also can crave the foods we grew up eating, or the foods

of our ancestors. This is one way that we seek comfort and familiarity. I know I have a special spot in my heart for spaghetti—a staple at my house since it was the only meal that my dad claimed to know how to cook.

Where you grew up can also have an impact on your eating preferences. Southerners take great pride in their barbecue, collard greens, and fried chicken. Chicagoans and New Yorkers get in heated debates about which city boasts the best pizza and hot dogs. Californians are known for their use of avocados and other fresh ingredients.

Your ancestry can also have an effect on your cravings. If you are Polish, you may crave pierogies; British and Irish people may crave fish and chips; and Italians may desire dishes that unite the classic flavors of tomato, cheese, and basil.

Incorporating the foods of our ancestors, regions, and childhoods into our diets on a regular basis can help us to meet those cravings. You may find that, during times of change and transition, you gravitate towards these familiar dishes. That is okay! Better yet, you can find healthier versions of those foods and recipes that still satisfy your cravings and share them with your community. Food is a wonderful tool for bonding with those around you, and sharing a part of you through food is a fun way to do it.

Life Imbalance

Another potential emotional trigger for cravings is life imbalance. When we feel unsatisfied in the various areas of our lives or we are out of balance in those areas, cravings can come. For instance, if you are a person who has a terrible job situation where you hate waking up every morning to go into the office, you feel stagnant, unsupported in your work and unappreciated; you may find that you use food to help. Maybe you munch on sugary or processed foods throughout the day, or maybe you have a free-for-all when you get home as a way to reward yourself for making it through the day.

Your career is just one area that can function this way. You may also feel trapped in an unhealthy relationship. Maybe you feel lost spiritually. It could also be that your finances have recently taken a hit. These are just a few areas of our lives that can affect our eating.

The remedy? Put down the fork and stop using food to dull your problems. Food just gives you a temporary distraction from what is really going on, but it doesn't solve anything. In fact, it adds to your problems if all the indulgent overeating puts on the pounds. Now you've got a weight and eating problem on top of the other stuff going on. Read on for more ideas on how to have a healthy response to your cravings.

Understanding Your Cravings

Now that you know that cravings are messages sent by your body to tell you that something is out of balance, it is your job to uncover what the root of the problem is and remedy the situation. As discussed above, there could be any number of things going on that are causing your cravings. A little detective work on your part is needed.

Probably the easiest first step is to decide if the cause of your craving is physical or emotional. Emotional triggers are a little bit easier to spot, so start there. In the moment you experience your craving, ask yourself:

- What am I feeling right now?
- Has anything happened that has affected my emotions?
- What's going on in my life that may be throwing me off balance?
- Am I under a lot of stress right now?

- Do I have enough excitement and variety in my life? When was the last time I had fun?
- Am I seeking comfort? Is what I am craving something from my past?
- How are my relationships?
- How is work?
- How is my spiritual life?

Through asking yourself these questions, you can discover if your craving has an emotional root. If nothing really stands out from this series of questions, you may have something more physical going on. To pinpoint a physical trigger, ask yourself these questions when your craving comes on:

- Has my diet been varied and based on healthy whole foods?
- Am I getting all of the essential nutrients that my body needs to perform at an optimum level?
- When was my last meal? Do I feel shaky, light-headed, or ravenous?
- Have I been drinking plenty of water today?
- Am I sleeping enough at night?
- How are my hormones? Am I at a particular point in my cycle or experiencing some other hormonal changes such as menopause or pregnancy?
- What season is it? Am I craving foods that are related to seasonality?
- Are the foods I am craving potentially addictive? Do I experience a "high" and "low" when I eat them?
- Are the foods I am craving high in fat or sugar?
- Have I been restricting my food choices in any way?

If any of these questions struck a chord, it is likely that your craving is physical, and you can approach it accordingly.

It is of course possible for your cravings to have several causes, from both physical and emotional triggers. Maybe you had another rough day at work, you haven't had much to eat or drink because you didn't have time, and you suddenly get a massive craving the moment you walk in the door at home. Emotionally, your job is probably not working well for you, and you are stressed. Physically, it is likely that you are dehydrated and have low blood sugar. Boom—a craving! It's pretty much inevitable. That does not mean though, that all hope is lost. There are simple, healthy ways to ward off cravings and also to respond to them when they do arise.

LINDSAY REINHOLT

20. FINDING A HEALTHY RESPONSE

Once you've figured out the cause (or causes) of your craving, you need to find a healthy and appropriate response. Really, when you think about it, giving into a craving for a donut when the cause of the craving is the fight you just had with your spouse is about as helpful as changing a light bulb by watching a movie (therefore, NOT!).

Your response needs to address the cause, and food does not do that. Once you've narrowed down what is causing your craving by asking yourself the questions above, you need to figure out how to respond to the cause. Maybe you can act immediately, and maybe you need to come up with a plan to implement over time, but try to do *something* right away.

If you are dehydrated, have a tall glass of water. Problem solved! If you are craving something from your youth, make a healthier version of it (best-case scenario), or have a small portion that still satisfies that craving (next-best-case scenario).

Bigger problems may not be as easily fixed, but doing something to progress to a solution will help you feel better and most likely calm that craving. For instance, if you hate your job, it's unlikely that you can find an immediate solution. Instead, you may need to consider some options for how to either to (a) find more satisfaction in your work and learn to enjoy it, or (b) look for alternative career options. Again, you are unlikely to find a fix immediately, but come up with a plan of action for how to address the specific issue in your life, rather than just dulling the problem with potato chips.

Repeat Cravings

Remember how we talked about how some people are self-described "sweet" people and others are "salty?" People often get cravings for specific foods repeatedly. One of the best ways to deal with cravings that you seem to get regularly is to sprinkle those foods throughout your eating schedule in healthy quantities, so that you never feel deprived. I love chocolate, so I enjoy having a small piece of dark chocolate one or two times a day. This helps me not to go crazy later on when I haven't gotten my chocolate "fix."

Boredom Eating

Are you a boredom eater? This is especially common for people who stay at home during the day, either for work or with kids. You also see it happen in the evening hours between dinner and bedtime, and on the weekends. You may not even be aware of the fact that you are bored. Maybe you are watching TV, and suddenly find yourself drifting into the kitchen to sneak a peak into the pantry. This kind of eating also happens during transitions. You just finished the laundry and before you get going on checking your email, you suddenly *need* a snack. If you suspect your cravings are the result of boredom, then find something enjoyable to do to distract yourself for twenty minutes, and then revisit the question of food. If even after engaging in a fun, stimulating activity you still think that you are hungry, then have something!

Stress Eating

Maybe stress sends you into an eating tailspin. I had a client who would use food to calm her when she would get overly stressed. Her vice was crackers—not shocking at all because the "crunch" of foods like crackers is shown to be quite pleasurable to humans. Psychologists actually believe that crunching can be cathartic—it helps us release our pent-up aggression. A simple solution to stress eating is to indulge in some self-care. Get a massage, read a guilty-pleasure book or a fun magazine, call up an old friend, take a hot bath, or get your nails done. It doesn't matter what it is, just do something for *yourself* that feels a little indulgent and special.

Restriction and Needing to Be Bad

The client who used crackers for stress relief often described her cracker episodes as an opportunity to "be bad." It sort of functioned as a mini-rebellion for her. If you spend most of your life playing by the "rules"—not only with food, but also in your personal, social, and professional lives—then you may seek an outlet where you can break free from that restriction.

Restriction can cause eating problems very early in life. I remember that when I was little, younger than 10 years old, we had a cookie jar that was always full of Oreos. I was only allowed to have them as a dessert after dinner, but having this rule in place just made them more attractive. I would sneak Oreos all the time, eating far too many when I could get my hands on them. Deprivation is not your friend, people!

The solution here is to find other ways to "be bad" as long as those choices wouldn't have any negative effects on you or others. People are imperfect. It is actually a *healthy* choice to admit it and allow imperfection in your life. You are living more authentically by doing so. Think about ways that you can "be bad" that may help to release some of that tension from trying to do everything perfectly. Say "no" to commitments you would normally agree to, sleep in, skip the gym, or buy yourself those shoes that you've been eyeing. Whatever sounds a little risky to you, but makes you feel a little freer. Again, try to add moments where you can be bad more regularly, so that you don't find yourself elbows-deep in a chocolate cake in an attempt to break the rules.

Trigger Foods

Maybe you have certain foods that, upon *seeing* them or *thinking* about them, you immediately want to *devour*. These are your trigger foods. Most people can come up with a few of their trigger foods on the spot. "Oh, Nutella is my weakness!" "I can't help myself around french fries!" Whatever your trigger foods may be, if they have an overly powerful hold on you and make it difficult for you to ignore them if they are around, then you may want to consider getting them out of your house, *at least for now*. Don't worry: It doesn't have to be a permanent thing. Usually, with less exposure, the pull of these foods weakens until they are no longer triggers for you, so you may be able to once again have them around in the future. For now, though, do yourself a favor and get rid of them.

Now, I'm not saying that you aren't allowed to eat these foods at all. Rather, if you find yourself craving, say a Snickers bar, and Snickers bars are a trigger for you, then you may want to set up some sort of system for how to handle that craving. For instance, if you want a Snickers bar, that is fine, but you have to get into the car and drive to the store to buy ONE, SINGLE-PORTION bar. Then when you go to eat it, you must concentrate on fully enjoying every bite. Afterwards, you can go back to whatever you were doing, knowing that you were able to satisfy that craving without going overboard. Plus, the fact that you have to leave your house to run an errand for one measly Snickers bar may be enough of a deterrent to keep you from eating it anyway. At the very least, you will probably check in with yourself to see if you *really* want it that badly.

Set Yourself Up for Success

Beyond just getting your trigger foods out of your house, there are several ways that you can set yourself up for success with food. It is much easier to adhere to your Goals and live your Intention if your environment is conducive to it.

Starting off first thing in the morning, have a balanced breakfast. Try to have all the macronutrients represented (carbohydrate, protein, and fat), and include some fiber. Some ideas include:

- A veggie and cheese omelet with an apple on the side
- Oatmeal with nuts and berries
- A green smoothie with kale, Greek yogurt, almond milk, and fruit
- Avocado toast with a couple eggs

When you start your day off with a complete healthy breakfast, your body immediately receives good fuel to get things going. Plus, the combination of fat, protein, and fiber will help to keep you satisfied for longer, making it less likely that you will experience the mid-morning munchies. You are also less prone to having cravings throughout the day because your blood sugar will be steadier.

Another way to set yourself up for success is to keep healthy snacks prepped and on hand. Have grab-and-go baggies of pre-made trail mix, single-serving containers of yogurt, celery cut and in a container with a scoop of peanut butter, plain popcorn, hummus and crackers, etc.—the list could go on and on. The key is to make your snacks accessible, portable, and already prepped. You are far more likely to eat something nutritious if it is easy to grab.

Did you know that alcohol can do a lot to mess with your cravings? For some people, a night with more than one drink can mess up food choices for the next several days and lead to more cravings. Plus, you are going to have a harder time fighting off those cravings if you are also dealing with a hangover, am I right? Be honest with yourself next time you have one too many and observe how it affects how you eat over the next couple of days. Consider tapering back your alcohol intake to help you to stay on track.

One way that I try to set myself up for success is to keep food out of sight. I work from home, so having a candy tray or other treats left out on the counter is a recipe for temptation for me. I can only resist for so long if I am constantly seeing something that sounds yummy. Even just moving it to the pantry makes it less appealing, less tempting. If I still need a treat, I know where to find it, but it isn't in my face all day long.

My last tip for setting yourself up to succeed is to spend more time away from the kitchen. My house is open-concept with a fairly small living space that really blends the kitchen into the family room. If I am in the family room, I am basically in the kitchen, with easy access to all the goodies I can find there. Because of this, I try to spend time in other areas of my house throughout the day, especially if I find food calling my name when I am not actually hungry for it. I go work for a bit in the office, play with my daughter in her room, or go down to the basement for some yoga and a change of venue. Do what works for you, but just know this: The closer you are to the kitchen, the more you will probably be thinking about food and eating, and the more likely it will be that you will find yourself eating when you aren't even hungry.

Remember Your Intention

In any of these cases, staying grounded in your Intention will give you focus for how to respond to the pull of food when you are not actually hungry. Remember that Intention Notecard? Next time you find yourself itching for food when you know that you aren't hungry, pull that out and read it. Keep it accessible so that you can always get to it quickly. Remind yourself of what your Intention is. Does eating in this moment or eating this particular food line up with your Intention? If not, it may be appropriate to rethink things and find something else to do.

If You Eat, Enjoy It

Lastly, if you find yourself craving something and none of the above techniques is working for you, it is okay to give yourself permission to eat. We are trying to get away from restriction, right? What I do ask is that if you do, be fully present for the entire eating experience. Really focus on the taste of every single bite of the food and enjoy it from start to finish. Sit down at the table, not on a sofa or in your car, and rid yourself of all distractions.

As you eat, check in with yourself regularly, and stop eating when you are satisfied. If you are fully engaged in the process and noticing the flavor of every bite, then you likely won't need as much to satisfy your craving.

Consider the Three Bite Rule with these sorts of cravings. The first bite is usually the best, the moment when the anticipation is finally rewarded with something delicious and decadent. The final bite is the grand finale, the last hurrah, the moment when you say good-bye to a wonderful dish that you have thoroughly enjoyed. All of the middle bites tend to be the same. If you just have three bites total, you get the entire, wonderful taste experience without all the unwanted calories. Not a bad gig, right?

21. MINDFUL EATING

This chapter is all about mindful eating. It is a continuation of Chapter Four: How We Were Meant to Eat, but I will expand here with some practical tools for how to actually achieve this yourself.

As a reminder, mindful eating is an approach that says that there is no right or wrong way to eat but rather that the goal is to be totally aware of the eating choices you make and why you make them. Eating should be based on hunger and nourishment, of both the body and soul, and you should be present during the entire eating experience. Furthermore, eating is a sensory experience in and of itself, and you should minimize outside distractions so that you can better focus on the food that you are consuming.

As discussed in Chapter Four, children are natural-born mindful eaters. Infants cry when they get hungry and happily drink milk until they are satisfied. Babies do not know how to overeat. They listen to their hunger and fullness and let it guide their eating. When children start consuming solid food, they spend a lot of time just exploring it—looking, feeling, smelling, and finally tasting it.

As we grow, we become more detached from the eating experience. We eat on the run and while doing other things like watching TV. We also stop paying attention to the food we put into our mouths. With mindful eating, the goal is to reconnect you with your inner childlike mindful eater.

Below, I have listed some tips to help you to start eating more mindfully, but don't get hung up on perfection. Mindfulness is like a muscle; it needs to be worked gradually to become strong. Maybe start with just one meal a day as you develop your mindful-eating practice. Over time, it will become more natural to where you can eat mindfully all of the time and do it without much effort at all.

Practice Gratitude

The first step in eating mindfully is to practice gratitude. We live during a time where food is very easy to access, and we are almost completely removed from the process that it took to get it to the store shelf. As you sit down to eat, say, an orange, think about the story of that particular orange. Imagine where it might have grown, what its tree looked like, who the farmer was who grew it and picked it. Imagine its journey from that farm to your local grocery store and all of the people who aided that journey from start to finish. Be thankful for all of the hands that went into bringing this delicious orange to you.

If you are eating something that is cooked, like a more complete meal, then you can approach it the same way. Whether you are eating out at a restaurant or at home, you can take a moment to think about the ingredients on your plate, where they came from, and who prepared them into this wonderful dish in front of you. Cooking really is an art form that should be appreciated before the dish gets devoured and disappears forever.

If you are spiritual, you can also include prayer as a way of expressing gratitude for the things in your life, including the food in front of you, recognizing that there are many blessings that you have for which you cannot take credit.

Eat With All Of Your Senses

Eating with gratitude naturally leads to a more sensory experience with food. As you pause to be grateful, you will notice the food in a whole different way than you would have if you had just jumped right in and started eating it. Eating mindfully means experiencing more than just the taste of the food: You approach the food utilizing *all* of your senses—sight, smell, touch, taste, and maybe even sound if it applies.

Sight

The first sense you will likely use is sight. As you sit down to eat your orange, you notice the coloring, shape, and the texture of it. You may even see a couple of imperfections that make this particular orange unique. Many foods, especially fruits and vegetables, are really quite beautiful. Phytochemicals are responsible for the colors in fruits and vegetables, and these disease-fighting nutrients are incredibly healthy for your body. Try to appreciate the colors on your plate, and work to get more of them into your meals. They are not only pretty to look at, but they are good for your body too!

If you go to a restaurant where the presentation of your food is thoughtfully considered, appreciate how the chef decided to plate your meal. It is believed that the appearance of food is as important as the taste by some chefs. Awards are even given out in culinary circles based on presentation alone. Have you ever watched a competition cooking show? If you have, then you know how plating can make or break a person's chance at winning any given cooking challenge.

Even if you don't go out often to restaurants, try bringing a little bit of presentation into your own home-cooked meals. You don't need a culinary degree or a ton of time to do this, either. Just play and experiment. Think of your food as art.

When you finish cooking, take a few extra moments to visualize how to arrange the food on the plate in a pleasing way. Use contrasting colors, make a design with the sauce or seasonings, put an odd (as opposed to even) number of items on the plate, add a simple garnish such as an herb sprig (parsley is cheap and looks great on everything), or use interesting utensils or dishes. You can't go wrong with white dishes, either—almost all food looks more appetizing on a white backdrop.

Smell

The next thing that you will probably notice soon after catching a glimpse of the food is its smell. Smells are especially captivating for us. They, more than any other sense, can trigger memories and emotions for humans. The olfactory bulb (the part of the brain that processes smells) is part of the limbic system. The limbic system is the part of the brain that deals with memory and emotion. It is because of this anatomical fact that smell is likely to be so closely related to memory and emotion.

The smell of warm cookies baking can immediately make you think of Christmastime with your mother preparing goodies in the kitchen. We wear perfume and cologne to attract others to us or to make us appear more appealing. The distinct smell of hospitals can draw up painful memories of times when you have seen someone close experience devastating health issues.

Pleasing smells can also elevate our moods. Have you ever woken up to the smells of eggs and bacon being cooked on the other side of the house? It probably made rolling out of bed a lot easier, didn't it?

A few years ago, my husband and I were looking to buy a house, and we met our realtor for a walk-through at a house that we were interested in. The first thing I remember noticing when we walked through the door was the warm, inviting smell of cranberries and cinnamon. The current owners had set up a candle warmer before they left that had been on long enough to fill the entire house with the rich, welcoming smell that immediately made the house feel like home. After leaving the walk-through, the first thing my husband commented on was not the excellent layout or nice appliances, but how good the house smelled! We ended up buying that house. Aroma matters!

In terms of mindful eating, make sure that you take a second (or a few seconds!) to appreciate the smell of your food. Enjoy the different smells through the entire cooking process if you were the one preparing the dish. I love the smell of garlic when I cook it in olive oil with some onions as the first step in many of the dishes that I like to prepare. As I'm cooking, I take a moment to get my nose right in the steam above the sauté pan as I stir the mixture. Even raw foods have great smells that you can enjoy. I use my sense of smell to pick out certain produce items at the store. Yep, I am *that* person that picks up cantaloupe after cantaloupe smelling each to find the sweetest one. Our noses were meant to be used to help us to find delicious and nutritious food in nature, so utilize yours!

A fun experiment for the next time you go to eat a dish prepared by someone else is to try to figure out what all is in it based on smell alone. Think about what the smell reminds you of and what individual smells you can detect as you inhale. Enjoy this step in the eating process without skipping over it.

Sound

Most people don't give much thought to the sense of hearing in regard to food. We don't think about food making sounds. Sure, maybe the cow mooed, but the steak on my plate isn't going to be making any noises by the time it reaches me. Or will it?

If you think about it, and start noticing, food does make noise—and it can be a whole symphony if you pay enough attention. Maybe your cereal "snaps, crackles, and pops" or your fajita meat and veggies are served on a skillet that is still sizzling. As you eat your food, it may make sounds as well—the crunch of a carrot or the subtle sound of your spoon going through chocolate mousse. A favorite for me is the crack of my spoon breaking through the glasslike sugar on top of crème brulee. I also love the sound of popping popcorn on the stovetop. It's so fun and sporadic, and connects me to my inner child.

As you start your practice of mindful eating, begin noticing the sounds of your food. Cooking usually makes all kinds of sounds and eating does as well. Scientists have found that the sound our food makes can greatly increase our enjoyment of that meal. Next time you eat anything, I challenge you to pay attention to the sounds the food gives off as well as the sounds you make when eating it—from the moment you start making it to the point you pop it in your mouth, chew, and swallow.

Touch

Next, part of eating is the sense of touch. If you are eating a burger, a wrap, a piece of fruit, some vegetables, or anything else for which you don't have to use a utensil, then you can use your sense of touch before the food even enters your mouth. Is the texture smooth or bumpy? Is the temperature warm or cool? Is the food hard or soft? All of these questions are answered the second you reach for the food item. Notice and enjoy how these foods feel between your fingers as they make their journey towards your lips.

If you use utensils, you won't feel the food until it crosses the threshold into your mouth. That's okay, though, because one of the most satisfying aspects of the sense of touch is what is called "mouthfeel." Mouthfeel basically means the texture you notice as you move the food around in your mouth—from the initial bite to your tongue and teeth moving it around and chewing, and then finally when you swallow it. How does the food feel inside your mouth?

If you think back over the foods that you have eaten in the past twenty-four hours, you probably can see that you have had a wide array of experiences with regard to mouthfeel. Creamy, crispy, gooey, brittle, sticky, silky, smooth, thick, chunky, chewy, grainy, etc.—all of these adjectives describe the mouthfeel of various foods.

Mouthfeel can be pleasant or unpleasant, depending on the person and the food. Part of the allure of chocolate for me is the fact that it melts in my mouth. It takes very little heat to turn it from solid to creamy liquid, part of the experience that I love and the reason why I enjoy eating chocolate so slowly. My husband, on the other hand, has an aversion to beans because of their mealy texture. You probably are already aware of some of the textures that appeal to you and turn you away, but spend more time experimenting with it. Instead of chewing just to get something swallowed, try to find pleasure in the chewing process, noting how the food feels inside of your mouth.

Taste

Finally, the grand finale of the sensory experience: tasting the food. When people think about their favorite foods and why they like them, taste is the first thing that is mentioned—and for good reason. Taste is probably the most obvious of the senses involved with food, but, unfortunately, many people don't fully appreciate all that it offers. They eat quickly, just trying to get through the food and on to the next thing on the agenda. Auto-pilot eating is also a regular occurrence, where a person gobbles through a whole meal only to realize they don't remember much about how it tasted.

These are symptoms of our hurried and stressed society. It's no wonder we have so many sick people! Reclaiming your mealtime and snack time is just one way that you can slow life down and enjoy it more. Taking the time to really experience the flavor of your food allows you to be present in the moment in a whole new way.

Next time you sit down to a meal, try this experiment. With each bite, try to pinpoint all of the flavors in your mouth. Trying to decipher all of the ingredients in a meal is a great way to get in touch with your sense of taste and can be a fun way to test your taste buds.

If you eat at home, the person who didn't cook the meal can take a stab at this exercise with the home cook able to tell them "yea" or "nay" on various ingredients. If you are out to eat, guessing all of the individual ingredients can help to give you an idea of how you might attempt to recreate the dish at home in the future.

A variation of this exercise that can be particularly fun is a Blindfolded Taste Test. With a partner, take turns creating "bites" of food for one another. The "taster" is blindfolded and the "cook" feeds them the bite, but not before describing both its mouthfeel (creamy, thick, crunchy, warm, etc.) and its general taste (sweet, salty, savory, etc.) The "taster" then gets to eat the bite, guessing what all was in it. Then, they switch roles. This is a great way to experience the flavor of a food because you are minimizing use of your other senses. You can use this exercise as a way to develop your palate or even a fun and cheap date-night activity.

A very practical way to do this all the time is to simply close your eyes for the first bite of each meal. You can then devote all of your attention to the food in your mouth and set the tone for a more mindful eating experience.

Chew More

One easy way to ensure that you really taste your food is to focus on chewing more. It may seem simple, but many people rush through this step, barely chewing their food enough to get it swallowed.

What does chewing properly look like? I like to recommend between twenty and thirty chews per bite. With some foods, especially really soft foods, this may be overkill, but it is a good place to start to retrain yourself to chew more. With meat and hard produce items, twenty to thirty chews may be what it really takes to get your food to a good point to be swallowed.

There are lots of good reasons to devote more time to the process of chewing. For one, chewing brings out more flavors in the food. As your teeth, tongue, and saliva work to break down the food, it releases even more flavors. If one of the things that you most love about food is the flavor (duh!), then it makes perfect sense to chew more. The longer you chew, the longer you get to experience that particular flavor. Who would want to rush through an experience like that?

Obviously, if you are devoting more time to chewing, it is going to take you longer to eat. This is a good thing! Slowing down allows you to enjoy the meal more, giving the food the respect and attention it deserves. Plus, it helps you to stay in touch with your body and its needs. Remember that it takes about twenty minutes for the brain to receive fullness signals from the gut? Give yourself at least that amount of time as you eat so that your brain has a fighting chance of getting the message before you go too far.

Remember, I am telling you that you are allowed, rather, *encouraged* to eat when you are hungry. Stopping a meal isn't a commitment to being done forever. You can always eat *whenever* you are hungry again, even if that is within the hour! Give yourself that permission, and putting your fork down when you are satisfied will become so much easier.

Next, chewing properly could ward off possible digestive issues. If you took anatomy or health class, then you may remember that digestion starts in the mouth. When you chew, enzymes in your saliva start breaking down the food right away and preparing it for better nutrient absorption. This makes it easier on the rest of your body to handle that food as it moves along. If you don't chew well, your gastrointestinal tract has to work a lot harder down the line to break that food down, which likely will cause some stomach discomfort and gas along the way. Not ideal, right? So, next time you are out to dinner on a date or with friends, remember to chew more, if only to avoid an embarrassing situation on the ride home.

There are several things you can do to slow down and start chewing better. Here are some tips to get you started:

- Remember the recommended minimum—twenty to thirty chews per bite.
- Give yourself plenty of time to enjoy your meal. Don't be rushed.
- Take smaller bites. They are easier to chew and force you to slow down.
- Put your fork down between bites.
- Wait until your food is completely swallowed before going back for another bite or a sip of your drink.
- Choose foods that take longer to eat. Crunchy foods can be more satisfying and force you to take your time more than softer foods.

Minimize Distractions

Chewing more will absolutely move you closer to eating mindfully, but there are some additional tricks you can use to slow down the eating experience.

As mentioned several times before, in order to properly practice mindful eating, you should do your best to minimize distractions during your meals. Turn off the television and put away your phone. Devote as much attention as possible to the food in front of you. Food is communal, so share your experience with anyone who may be eating with you. Talk about the food, where it came from, how it was prepared, what it tastes like, and the things that you enjoy about it. If you are eating alone, think about all of those same aspects of your food. Savor the opportunity for a quiet moment just to be present.

If you were the cook, honor the time that you gave to putting the food on the table. Don't just eat through it without a thought! If someone else made it, take a moment to appreciate the time and energy that they put into a delicious meal that you can now enjoy.

If you are eating with others, then save any serious, potentially confrontational conversations for another time. Eating when you are upset or tense will absolutely affect the taste of your food as well as your digestion of it. Maybe your food will improve how you are feeling, which would be wonderful, but don't let a bad mood ruin your good food. Just like the saying, "Never go to bed angry," I would like to offer the suggestion, "Never eat while angry." You are more likely to make poor eating choices, chew hastily, and have digestive issues afterwards. Try your best to come to your meals in a pleasant or at least neutral mood.

Simple Steps to Elevate the Eating Experience

My next suggestion is to, whenever possible, attempt to elevate your eating experiences. Eating is fun, health-promoting, indulgent, communal, sensory, and necessary. You've got to eat, so why not make your meals feel a little more special? There are simple, quick, and inexpensive ways to bring your eating experience to the next level, which will likely help you to enjoy your meal even more.

1. Sit down and eat at the table.

My first suggestion, at the risk of sounding like a broken record, is to *sit down* at the table to eat. I know that I've mentioned this a couple of times before, but that is because it is such a simple thing that makes such a big difference in what you choose to eat, how you go about eating that food, how much food you consume when all is said and done, and your enjoyment of the experience overall. Here we are talking about that final point—your enjoyment of the experience.

Imagine the difference between grabbing a breakfast-to-go as you run out the door and having enough time to sit down and eat something at home. First of all, you are going to have to choose something portable if you are eating in the car, so maybe you choose a breakfast bar. It's probably not all that unhealthy and most likely has several nutritional claims on its packaging like "No High Fructose Corn Syrup!" and "7 Grams of Protein Per Serving!" Those claims are all well and good, but they are probably on the label to distract you from the fact that it is a processed food, it's likely full of sugar, and it probably contains several ingredients that you can't even pronounce.

Next, let's look at *how* you are going to eat it. You will probably tear into that sucker as you pull out of your driveway, and chomp away as you turn, change lanes, and navigate your way all using your one free hand. Your attention will be on the traffic around you, maybe on your music on the radio, and definitely on the day ahead at work. You know what it won't be on? That's right, your breakfast bar. And maybe that's not a bad thing. It probably doesn't taste *that* good anyways.

Luckily, with the example of a breakfast bar, it is unlikely that you will overeat. On the other hand, if this same example was with something like a bag of chips, this mindless eating approach would likely lead to overeating. You just aren't paying enough attention to know when to stop.

Lastly, there is the question of enjoyment. Go back to your imagined drive to work with your breakfast bar. Do you think that you would have a positive, a negative, or a neutral attitude toward that eating experience when you thought back over it after the fact? Better yet, do you think you *would* think about it, ever again? Probably not. It wasn't an event worthy of memory.

Contrast that with a morning where you plan for enough time to prepare a meal to enjoy while sitting at the table. For this meal, let's imagine you are having some eggs, toast, and berries. It probably takes you all of five, maybe ten, minutes to whip this up, and you sit down to your meal. First of all, *what* you've chosen to eat is much less processed and much more of a complete meal. You are having a good mix of protein, carbs, fat, and fiber that is going to give your body the fuel it needs to kick off the day. It will help stabilize your blood sugar, so you will feel satisfied and not get hungry for several hours. Another huge bonus—it's warm! There is nothing like a warm, freshly cooked meal to start your day.

So, you've not only chosen a warm breakfast that is better for your body, but think about all of the attention you've freed up by not having the distraction of driving while eating! Sitting at the table, you can fully immerse yourself in your meal, enjoying the first moments of your day in a comforting and calm way. You are able to taste the food, which, let's be honest, will be so much more delicious than some crummy breakfast bar.

Do you get what I'm saying here through this example? Have I beaten the dead horse enough? Eat sitting down, at a table, whenever possible!

2. Consider the dishes

It may seem secondary, but *what* you choose to serve your food *on* is an important part of the eating experience. Sure there is a time and a place for plastic utensils and paper plates, but this should not be the norm. Using dishes that appeal to you or ones that make food look more appetizing can bring the whole dining experience to a new level. Remember that, after taste, sight is one of the most important senses involved with eating. If your food looks interesting, even beautiful, and at least appealing, then you are more likely to enjoy the taste of it too.

White plates are universally recognized for making food look good. They are simple, timeless, elegant, and expensive-looking, and they offer good contrast against the colors of the food. Plus, they look appropriate in all situations—formal or casual. I definitely recommend investing in some simple white dishes. You'll thank me years down the road when they haven't gone out of style and still make your food look amazing.

Another fun option is to keep your eye out for unique dishes that you can use for special occasions. I love antique teacups and saucers. Some people have a soft spot for coffee mugs or pint glasses. As a wedding gift, we were given a "tasting party" set that included all kinds of teensy dishes—small bowls, spoons, martini glasses that are four-inches high, and so on. I love using these for food prep, optional garnishes to bring to the table, or small side dishes, like berries.

Utensils shouldn't be neglected either. For instance, I cook a lot of Asian-inspired dishes, so we have several pairs of chopsticks that we like to pull out for such occasions. My toddler even has a set of training chopsticks with a cat on the top!

Don't forget about your drinks. Functionality is important, yes, but your beverage containers are also worthy of consideration. I have several friends who strongly prefer a stemmed wine glass to a stem-less one. Wine enthusiasts claim that the stem-less glasses affect the temperature of the wine, and that the bowl gathers debris by sitting directly on whatever surface you leave it. The people I know that prefer stemware, though, do so less for those reasons, and more for the experience of drinking the wine from a stemmed glass versus a stem-less one. The stemmed glass says, "I may have just spent the last two hours chasing kids around the house, burning the dinner, and folding the laundry, but I deserve a little elegance in my day." That's a pretty big statement from a skinny glass column that is only a few inches long!

On the front end of the day reside the caffeinated beverages. For most people, a cup of java in the morning is the ticket to getting them out of bed and on with their day. For others, tea offers a nice alternative. Either way, investing in some mugs that you love is a must. They don't have to be expensive either. For one thing, mugs are one of the few types of dishes that don't have to match. Sure, you can get a nice set that coordinates, but having a variety of mugs with different designs is especially helpful if you are serving a crowd. Everyone can tell their mug from the rest when it gets left on a table for a few minutes.

I also think mugs make great souvenirs. One of my favorite mugs is from this quirky coffee shop called the Smelly Cat Coffeehouse in Charlotte, North Carolina. It is a handmade ceramic mug with blue glaze and says, "Smelly Cat Coffeehouse." Plus, the handle is big so I can get my whole hand inside of it, which is necessary for me with any good mug. Another bonus is there is a little flat addition on the top of the handle where you can place your thumb—genius. One thing is certain: Whoever designed this mug is obviously a coffee lover.

My intention here is simply to inspire you to spend some time thinking about your dishes and how they add to or maybe detract from your eating and drinking experiences. Think about incorporating some of the things that I've suggested here, or finding your own ways to elevate your meals with different dishes.

3. Set the mood

Whether you are having a romantic dinner or not, setting the mood during your meal is a crucial component to how much you will enjoy it. Sure, you typically think of candles and dim lights for date night, which is great, but what about all of the other meals? Should environment be ignored in these settings? I think not!

All restaurant owners give consideration to the dining environment, from the lighting and décor to the music they choose to play in the background. To be certain, some are more successful at this than others. At your own home, try to think a little like a restaurant owner. What do you want the experience to be like for diners? How can the lighting, seating, and sounds help you to achieve the desired experience?

At our house, we've got a toddler who certainly steals the show during most of our meals. Despite that, we always try to sit down for dinner at the table, turn on some music that we all enjoy, and say a prayer of thanks for the food in front of us. When we think of it, we also light a candle.

Do what works and makes sense for you and your family, but

always be looking for ways to set the mood for a better meal with those around you.

22. WHOLE FOODS

In this chapter, we will continue the conversation from Chapter Two: What We Were Meant to Eat. We live during a time of nutrition information overload. You can't turn on the news, watch a talk show, read a magazine, or surf the Internet without being bombarded with food science. "Eat this! Not that!" "Protein is the most important macronutrient!" "Avoid animal fat!" "We should all avoid gluten!" "Make sure to eat your whole grains!"

Food experts and scientists are on quite a pedestal in our culture. We love listening to the latest and greatest "research" (or fad) that comes out in the media, and we love outsourcing our eating decisions to these people.

But, have you noticed that most of this "science" is in conflict? That's because nutrition is an ever-evolving science. We are really just starting to understand how food acts in the body. All the time new studies come out that disprove previous studies. Can you imagine if you abided by every suggestion that you ever heard about how to eat? You'd be constantly switching gears, throwing out certain food items, and buying new ones to take their places. It's enough to make your head spin.

On top of that, most of this food science is pretty hard to trust. Not because the scientists and researchers are untrustworthy and malicious, but mainly because it is really hard to study nutrition. For one, nutrition and digestion are incredibly complicated. It is not as simple as adding an input and looking for a reaction. There are too many moving parts with food, too many nutrients at play, reactions, and other components that have an effect on how food operates within the body.

Plus, most of these types of studies don't take into consideration other factors, such as lifestyle choices, family history, or an individual's metabolic rate.

Human beings as test subjects are inherently problematic for these reasons. Studies that have people self-report on what their diet is like cannot be trusted, either. Time and time again, we see that self-reporting leads to unreliable data because people aren't good at being accurate about what they have eaten. Especially in terms of quantity—they almost always underestimate the number of calories they consume.

Furthermore, there are just not enough studies that do a good job looking into the long-term effects of diet. Most of them only last a few months, which is hardly enough time to get meaningful data. There are a few studies that have been more long-term and collected decades of data. You may have heard of the Nurses' Health Studies, probably the most well known long-term studies, which started in 1976 and have analyzed the diets and lifestyles of 238,000 female nurses. These studies are remarkably still going on. Despite the very long-term nature of this work, the studies still rely on self-report and don't do enough to account for individual differences in the participants.

So what do you do in the wake of all this "research" that, in many ways, leads to more questions than answers? I believe that we should take a step back from every little report and study.

Sure, be informed. There is a difference between being informed and being a believer, though. If you believe every suggestion, then you are ultimately left with two options:

(a) try to apply it to your life, only to have to constantly change your diet because the research is conflicting; or

(b) feel so overwhelmed by all of the information out there that you feel paralyzed, so you just keep eating all the junk that everyone else is eating.

So instead of believing every little thing that you hear about nutrition, you have an alternative. You can choose to take back the control over your food that you have outsourced to "experts" for too long. Go back to the inherent knowledge that you were born with. People for generations living all over the world have lead healthy lives (with much lower incidence of lifestyle diseases, I might add) without the tinkering of scientists in their diets.

In a world of nutrition-information overload and general confusion due to that abundance of information, a simple answer exists. That answer is this:

Eat when you are hungry, and stop when you are full. Listen to your body and what it needs. Lastly, as often as possible, fill your diet with whole, natural foods.

We've discussed the hunger and satiation piece of that puzzle, as well as the tuning in with your body and what its signals mean for you. This chapter is all about the last part— eating whole, natural foods.

As a review, whole foods are foods that are as close to their natural form as possible. They are unprocessed, or very minimally processed, and have only one to maybe a few ingredients. All of the ingredients in whole foods are recognizable and pronounceable and don't sound like something from your high school chemistry class. "Clean" is another word used to describe this category of edibles. Fruits, vegetables, meats, nuts, whole grains, legumes, and minimally processed dairy all qualify as whole foods.

One of the best things about basing your diet on whole foods is that it takes the anxiety out of shopping, meal-preparing, and eating. With all of the information and "science" out there dictating how you should be eating, you can breathe a sigh of relief knowing that you can rise above all of the noise and just eat in a way that makes sense for you, your lifestyle, and your body. You don't have to feel stressed if you don't know everything there is to know about nutrition (no one does!) or if the science seems to constantly be changing (it is!). You just get to eat foods that you like, that your body will respond well to, and that are simple to find and prepare.

Another benefit to a whole-foods-based diet is that there is no math or magical formulas to follow. You don't have to worry about how many grams of protein versus carbs versus fat your meals have, how many calories you've got left to make it through the day, or how you will manage social events. Whole foods tend to be lower in calories than processed foods because they don't have as many added sugars and other ingredients that spike the calorie total. You are also more likely to get full more quickly when eating whole foods because they tend to have more fiber. Think corn on the cob versus high-fructose corn syrup or whole grain wheat bread versus Wonder Bread.

We've discussed what whole foods *are* at length, but let's take a closer look at which foods are *not* considered "whole." As I mentioned in Part One, if a whole food has an ingredient list, it reads like a recipe, not a science experiment. Therefore, non-whole foods are the ones that have long ingredient lists (my general cut-off is more than five ingredients) with ingredients that sound like chemicals. If you cannot pronounce an ingredient, can't picture what it looks like, or have no idea how to go about finding it at the store, then it probably isn't a whole food. Monosodium glutamate, lecithin, modified food starch, and calcium disodium EDTA are examples of ingredients to avoid if you are seeking a whole foods approach to your diet.

One of the problems with non-whole or *processed* foods is that we frankly don't know enough about how the human body responds to them. They haven't been around for that long. It is still unclear what the effect of all these additives and preservatives will be on long-term health. What is clear though, is that the Standard American Diet both is high in processed foods and is one of the leading causes of cancer, diabetes, heart disease, and other lifestyle-related diseases. Processed foods and these health issues go hand-in-hand. Sure, there are other contributors to the health epidemic that we face as a country, but it's enough to make me raise an eyebrow on the issue of processed foods.

When it comes down to it, doesn't it just make more sense to eat what we were meant to eat, not what some food scientist concocted in the lab? The truth is, food companies are not interested in your health. They are interested in making money, and, to do that, they utilize all of their resources to invent foods that are tasty and cheap. The best way to do that is to use cheap products and reformulate them into ingredients that they can use to increase flavor and shelf life. Bada-bing, bada-boom, and magically you've got Twinkies!

If you are used to regularly eating processed foods, it is likely that eating whole foods will take some getting used to. It takes a little more effort in the kitchen, probably some trial and error, and also trying a variety of foods to see what you like and what can work as substitutes for your previous choices.

The more you commit to this new lifestyle, though, the more you will reap the benefits. You will start feeling more energized and vibrant, and it is likely that you will lose weight. You will probably also notice that your taste buds start to change. The processed foods you used to enjoy will no longer taste as good to you. You may even be able to notice a chemical taste to some of them. Not yummy!

A Final Thought on Whole Foods Versus Processed Foods

Although I clearly am in favor of a whole-foods-based diet, I also spent a lot of time in this book advocating against deprivation. Yes, many experts including me believe that the human body thrives best when consuming whole foods, but there is also something to be said for flexibility. You should embrace all foods as just food, not moral obligations to choose the right or wrong ones. You cannot ignore the facts, though, that some foods function in the body and serve us better than others do. Just use the knowledge you have gained here to inform your eating decisions and try to choose whole foods *most of the time*. Remember that it is not about 100-percent perfection. One meal, one day, one vacation, and so on, isn't going to bring destruction to your health and happiness. Dust yourself off, remind yourself of why you choose to eat this way, and then go make yourself a kale and berry smoothie.

23. BRANCH OUT IN THE KITCHEN

If you are serious about nurturing your relationship with food and improving your health, then spending time in the kitchen is not negotiable. In order to minimize processed food and maximize whole foods, you have got to learn how to prepare your own meals.

Maybe you consider yourself a master chef, or maybe you think your cooking expertise is limited to reheating meals in the microwave. Wherever you are on that spectrum, there is always room for improvement. In this chapter, I am going to outline some tips on how to branch out in the kitchen and become a better cook. I will also discuss the importance of expanding your food choices and being open to new flavors. The culinary landscape is vast and interesting. You could easily spend a lifetime exploring it. Get excited to start learning new techniques and trying foods you've never had before.

Become a Mindful Cook

First and foremost, to become a better cook, you should become more mindful. We've talked about mindfulness in eating, but now we are applying it to cooking. Mindfulness is about being in the present moment and having a higher level of awareness. Sometimes you may feel rushed to get something on the table, but the tension with which you cook will absolutely come through in your final meal. Instead, light a candle, put on some music that you enjoy, and take a breath before you start cooking. Set up your space so that you have plenty of room to work, and make sure everything is clean before you get started.

Just like when you eat, use all five senses as you cook. Look at the food as it cooks to gain clues about how close it is to being done. Smell the aromas coming off of the ingredients as they change due to the heat. Listen for the sounds that the foods make as they sizzle, steam, and char. Touch your food to check for doneness. If you don't know about it already, learn more about how the doneness of steak can be checked by comparing the feel of the steak to different parts of your hand. Lastly, taste and season your food throughout the cooking process. Adding seasoning too early or too late can result in a less-flavorful meal.

Constantly be modifying as you go. Remember, recipes are written by humans who are not perfect and do not have the same taste preferences as you do. Leave some wiggle room wherein you can modify the recipes that you make to create something that is your own.

Simple Ways to Become More Efficient in the Kitchen

Even though you may be spending more time preparing food than you are used to, there are some great ways to become more efficient with your time.

1. When it Makes Sense, Choose Convenience

First, you can cut down on the time it takes to cook before you even leave the grocery store. Consider choosing ingredients that are ready-to-go, such as bagged pre-shredded lettuce and pre-diced onions. Yes, these tend to be more expensive per ounce than their non-prepped counterparts, but sometimes it is worth paying for the convenience. It often also makes sense to purchase healthy "convenience" foods and keep stocked up. For instance, canned tomatoes and tomato paste are staples at our house for making sauces and soups. Frozen fruits and vegetables are great since they won't rot and you can use them whenever you need them. They also retain more nutrients than canned produce items, so you get a little more nutritional bang for your buck!

2. Prep Ahead

If you choose to buy foods that are not pre-prepared, then prep them immediately when you get home from the store. When I buy lettuce, I immediately wash, tear, and dry it in a spinner. Then I store it in large plastic bags with a piece of paper towel to soak up the extra moisture. This not only helps it stay fresh longer, but also means that all I have to do when I need lettuce is to pour it into a bowl. Needless to say, we eat many more salads when I have lettuce already prepared in this way. You can do this with many of your produce purchases without making them rot sooner. It is also a good idea to make snack packs with nuts, dried fruit, dried coconut, and other ingredients so that you have healthy, single serving snacks ready to go at a moment's notice.

3. Cook Once, Eat Twice (Or More)

Another tip to become more efficient in the kitchen is to cook once and eat many times. Probably the most obvious way to do this is to cook so that you have leftovers. If you have a fairly small family (one or two members), you can probably get by through simply cooking recipes as they are written, and you will have plenty of leftovers as a result. If your family is larger, though, then you may want to consider doubling your recipes to ensure some is leftover for future meals.

Another useful tip is to store your leftovers in small, single-serving, glass containers. That way, when someone goes to eat it, they can just get out the one container and a meal is ready to go. Plus, if you are in a crunch (or you just don't want to dirty more dishes) you can heat and eat out of the same container it was stored in. Pretty efficient, huh?

4. Repurpose

Leftovers are great, but there are some other choices you can make that will save you cooking time. When you make a dish that calls for some sort of cooked grain, such as rice or quinoa, double the batch. Store the leftovers in the fridge, and you've got easy side dishes and salad additions for the rest of the week. Grains are incredibly versatile, so think outside of the box. Rice isn't just an accompaniment to Asian main courses but can also be used in breakfast, like rice porridge, and dessert, such as rice pudding. Same thing goes for quinoa, oats, etc. Find fun recipes for repurposing your grains.

Repurposing works for more than just grains. One thing that can save you both time and money (win-win!) is to buy meat in large quantities when it is on sale. Then, take it home and cook it up. For instance, buy a large pack of chicken breasts and grill or bake them right away. Suddenly, you've got protein for salads, soup, stir-fry, tacos, pasta, sandwiches, pizza, curry, chicken salad, casseroles, etc.—the possibilities are endless! I also like to keep my eye out for large cheap cuts of meat, such as shoulder or round roasts. I throw these in the slow cooker, and they get super tender and yield a ton of meat to use for all kinds of things. Can anyone say "pot roast" or "pulled pork"? How about "carnitas"?

5. Utilize Your Gadgets

You can also put your kitchen appliances to work for you to

make your job easier. Like I just mentioned, the slow cooker can be your best friend for turning a cheap, tough cut of meat into something delicious and juicy. Slow cookers can also free you from the kitchen—you really can set it and forget it!

Most slow cooker recipes just require dumping a few ingredients into the pot, setting the heat, and walking away. Then, after a long day at work when the last thing you feel like is cooking dinner, you walk in the door to the warm, savory aromas of a dinner *that cooked itself.* And it's even easier if you use a slow cooker liner to make clean up a breeze!

Another beautiful thing about slow cookers is that you don't need a recipe to use them. As a rule of thumb, just put these items in your slow cooker in order: vegetables, protein, spices, and liquid. Set the heat to low or high, depending on how long you have to cook it, and walk away!

Lastly, you can devote a few hours one day to prepping lots of slow-cooker meals, store them in a plastic freezer bag, and then pull one out whenever you want. All you have to do is thaw the bag in the fridge overnight and dump its contents into your slow cooker the next day. Voila! Dinner is done! There are tons of great resources on the Internet for this kind of meal prep—I highly recommend that you look into it. You'll thank me later.

Similar to your slow cooker, your freezer can also become a handy, time-saving appliance. As mentioned above, you can store prepped slow cooker meals in the freezer for use whenever you want. You should also get comfortable with storing leftovers in the freezer if you don't think you will have a chance to eat them before they spoil in the fridge. Most foods do well frozen and then reheated, especially if you give them time to thaw in the fridge. When I make stock or pesto, I always make extra so that I can freeze it in ice-cube trays and pop out a cube whenever I want for the recipes that I am preparing. If you grow your own herbs in the summer, you can also freeze clippings of those herbs, plus a little oil or water in ice-cube trays to thaw in future recipes. When certain foods are in season, such as berries, you can freeze them to make pies, jams, or smoothies in the winter. Learn to love your freezer—just make sure that you check it regularly so that you don't forget what's in there.

Try New Techniques

No matter where you are on the spectrum of cooking know-how, you can always learn some new techniques. If you are starting from nothing, get really comfortable with baking and cooking on the stove. Look for recipes with "easy" in the title. Plus, if you are cooking with clean, whole foods, you are more likely to find simple recipes that don't take too much effort.

If you feel pretty comfortable with the oven and stove, then branch out a bit. Maybe consider different ways of preparing your vegetables. Common ones include sautéing and roasting, but there are many other options. Steaming vegetables is probably the healthiest as it helps to retain more of the vegetables' nutrients that are lost through other cooking methods. You can also try blanching or even grilling your vegetables for fun alternatives.

Learn how to use different appliances for cooking your foods. Many women leave the grilling work to their husbands, but it is worth getting familiar with the grill, even if you only use it every once in a while. Food dehydrators are inexpensive and really easy to use. They give you a means to preparing all kinds of delicious snacks that keep really well. We like making beef jerky and dried apple and banana chips with ours. A smoker is also a fun tool for cooking meat. The process takes several hours, but it is fairly easy and turns meat into heavenly deliciousness. Fermentation may sound scary but it is absurdly easy and a really healthy way to prepare food. You can make kimchi, sauerkraut, or kombucha. Do a little research, and you'll be on your way to all of the wonderful health benefits of fermented foods. Lastly, canning can be a great way to use up the produce you can get in excess in the summer and make it last through the coming winter. It takes a little learning and investment in some equipment, but is really easy once you do that initial work.

Get Geared Up: Equipment

You can't cook properly without the right equipment. Hopefully you've got the basics, such as pots, pans, cooking utensils, oven, and stove. Depending on the quality of those items, you may want to think about upgrading to nicer ones, especially if you think that it would help you to cook more often and to enjoy the process more. Non-stick cookware is a must, as are a few wooden spoons, some tongs, and LOTS of spatulas. I seem to use spatulas like crazy, so I like to have many on hand so I don't run out before I get the chance to run the dishwasher.

There are several items that aren't mandatory but certainly make your life easier in the kitchen. One of the tools that I find especially helpful is an instant-read digital meat thermometer. Ovens vary in temperature, and some recipes simply have incorrect cook times. It's handy to have a thermometer to check the internal temperature of your cooked meat, so that you KNOW for certain that it is cooked through and aren't tempted to overcook it just to be sure.

I also find that having lots of little bowls for prepped ingredients helps to streamline the cooking process. When a sautéed kale recipe calls for "1 bunch kale, torn into bite-sized pieces" to be added to oil and garlic after the garlic has cooked for a couple minutes, it is helpful if you have the kale already torn before you even start the recipe by turning on the stove. Otherwise, you will likely neglect the cooking garlic while you frantically tear kale, trying to get it in before the garlic is overcooked. Plus, the garlic will probably be unevenly cooked, maybe even burned, from not being stirred. With small prep bowls, you can measure out all of your ingredients and chop, dice, shred, or whatever you are supposed to do, *before* you start the actual cooking process. Then you can just dump in the ingredients at the designated times along the way. This technique also frees you up to *taste as you go*, something that we discussed in the section about becoming a mindful cook.

Small bowls are great for prep, but it is also nice to have a big bowl to use as your garbage bowl. Take a note from Rachel Ray, and use this bowl to throw all of the vegetable scraps, packaging, and other trash items that accumulate as you cook. This helps you to stay at your station as you cut and prep, instead of going to and from the garbage can all the time.

You probably have a cutting board or two, but I would suggest having several. Glass cutting boards are the worst, so stay away from them all costs. Wooden or plastic cutting boards are much better for cutting, and they don't slip as often. As you do your meal prep, make sure to cut vegetables before you use the cutting board for any raw meat. That way, you keep things sanitary and don't have to use more than one cutting board per meal.

Get Geared Up: Food

If you are trying to become more efficient in the kitchen, it is obligatory that you keep a well-stocked pantry and refrigerator. It gets tedious to have to run to the grocery store every time you set out to make a meal. Keep staples on hand all the time. At our house, I try to always have several types of grains, such as brown rice, quinoa, oats, and noodles, in the pantry. I also keep diced tomatoes and tomato paste for making sauces and adding to recipes. It is also important to have a variety of vinegars and oils because they come up in recipes all of the time. Obviously, having the most common herbs and spices is also helpful. Ones that we use frequently are garlic powder, chili powder, onion powder, basil, oregano, parsley, paprika, cinnamon, ginger, cumin, salt, and pepper. Since I cook a lot of Asian food, we always keep soy sauce, fish sauce, and curry paste in our fridge. Find the things you like or use frequently in the meals you prepare and stock up. Also, when you run out of these items, immediately add them to your grocery list. Otherwise, you may find yourself cooking soup without any chicken stock in the pantry.

Practice Makes Perfect

Cooking is a skill that takes practice. The more experience you have preparing food in different ways, the more efficient and easy it will become. Plus, you will become increasingly familiar with your taste preferences and so will get better at choosing recipes and making up meals as you go.

My husband's grandmother is a wonderful cook. She is known for her yeast rolls and monster cookies in particular. I always loved eating her food, but when I would ask how she made some of her dishes, I would become lost with her response. "Oh a little of this, a little of that" was sort of what I would get. But what about the precise measurements for everything? I needed a full ingredient list at the beginning followed by clear, sequential instructions.

Now, I totally get it. I have found that the more years I have added to my cooking experience, the more comfortable I have become with "winging it." There are many meals that I make that I would have a darn hard time writing out a recipe for. In all reality, these dishes come out slightly different every time. I can cook a fantastic coconut curry fish dinner, but don't you dare ask me how I make it. I'm not sure I could really describe it well enough and guess on the amounts of all the ingredients accurately. I know what it looks and tastes like through each step of the cooking process, and that's enough for me to make it.

I like cooking this way. It's fun, and even therapeutic to me. It makes me feel powerful and imaginative. I created something, and it is delicious! If I do use a recipe, I frequently deviate from it to suit my tastes, time frame, cooking method preference, and the ingredients I have available. I know what I like and what works together.

This wasn't always the case. It is a product of practice, and I look forward to seeing where the years ahead take me and my culinary skills. You can develop your skills in the kitchen too. You just have to put in the time. Say it with me: "Practice makes perfect!"

Try New Foods

How you cook isn't the only way that you should branch out. Another important way to develop your relationship with food is in *what* you choose to cook and eat. Life is too short to eat the same food over and over again. Our palates, and our bodies really, need variety! One of the easiest areas to explore on your own is produce. Of the over 20,000 known edible plants on this planet, less than twenty of them constitute ninety-percent of our diets.[9] That leaves a lot of room for exploration! Passion fruit, blood oranges, star fruit, radicchio, swiss chard, okra, and baby bok choy are all fruits and vegetables you can probably find at your local grocery store. Explore the produce section next time you go for a grocery run, and find something new. I often recommend to my clients to try a new plant each week. You may come up against some that you don't like, but you are bound to find some new favorites, as well. You can't know unless you try!

I also love trying new foods when I travel. My husband and

I always say that one of our favorite ways to explore a new city is to "eat our way through it." Eating the way the locals eat is one of the best ways to immerse yourself in a culture, plus it's a lot of fun. You are going to have to eat while you travel, so you may as well make it part of the experience. Before you go somewhere in particular, do a little light research on what dishes and drinks they are known for. Southern barbecue is the best, you can't beat eating lobster on the coast of Maine, and there's nothing like paella on the Mediterranean in Spain.

Even if something seems weird or flat-out disgusting, I highly recommend that you try it if it is typical to the area where you are. At a bed and breakfast in England, our breakfasts were served with black pudding. If you aren't familiar with the dish, let me start by saying it in NO WAY resembles what Americans call pudding. Rather it is a kind of blood sausage made from a mixture of pork fat, blood and oatmeal or grits, depending on the recipe. When it came out on my plate, it was a dark-black square, similar in texture to a very dense, moist brownie. I knew what was in it, but I tried it anyways. I gagged a bit at the taste, and I will probably never eat it again, but I am glad I can now say that I've tried black pudding. That's what life is about.

Share What You've Learned With Your Loved Ones

Cooking and eating should not be solo experiences. Sure, there are going to be meals that you eat alone, but, for the most part, eating is social. As you've made your way through the suggestions in this book, you've likely started developing new tastes and skills that those around you would benefit from experiencing themselves. Don't hold back on sharing what you've learned with them. Invite your friends and families into the kitchen with you.

Next time you invite someone over to your place for a meal, ask them to come early to share in the meal prep. Instead of turning Netflix on for your kids while you prepare the family dinner, have them join you in the kitchen and give them age-appropriate tasks to help. It is my belief that one of the most valuable skills and passions that you can pass down to your children is the art of cooking. Teach them to love it and care about what they eat and how it is prepared. Their future health and happiness will likely be much greater for your taking the time to model this behavior now. Plus, as they get older, you will probably have some very capable sous chefs working with you as you put meals together.

Besides the cooking process, share new foods with those around you. Don't always play it safe. Try cooking unique foods or meals from another cuisine when you have friends or family over. Better yet, host a theme night! You can base it on cuisine, such as Moroccan, Irish, or Japanese, and have everyone bring something different that relates. Another option is to pick an ingredient to feature in each course. For instance, you could choose pomegranate and have a starter salad that features pomegranate seeds and goat cheese. For the main dish you could do meat with a pomegranate sauce, such as lamb or chicken. Dessert could be a delicious pomegranate apple crisp. Sounds fun, right?

It doesn't really matter how you choose to share cooking and food with your loved ones. No matter what you do, you will see everyone benefit. Everyone's skills and palates will expand as you try preparing and tasting new dishes. Sharing new experiences is a great way to bond, which will grow your relationships. By trying new things, you are inviting others into the mindful-eating experience, where they are focusing more on all five of their senses during the meal. The list goes on and on.

24. PUTTING IT ALL TOGETHER

We have come to the end of this book, but it is certainly not the end of your journey. The job is not yet done; we are all works in progress. At this point, you hopefully have acquired a new skillset, one that will steer you ever closer toward a healthy relationship with food.

I read once about a scientist that claimed he had solved the world's health and food crisis by developing a "meal" that was made up of all of the nutrients our bodies need in the perfect proportions. It wasn't even really food, but rather a mixture of protein, carbohydrate, fat, fiber, vitamins, and minerals concocted in a lab. The scientist claimed it was the silver bullet—no more obesity or its related health problems. In addition, there would be an end to starvation in areas where food was scarce. Plus, people wouldn't be burdened with the constant decision of what to eat and the subsequent preparation of the chosen food. They would simply tear open their miracle meal packs, fuel up, and continue about their days. I remember thinking about how sad this notion was, that food was simply a means to one end: physical survival.

Food is so much more than the sum of its nutrients, and eating is so much more than putting food in your mouth and chewing. It is a pleasure, a political statement, a social endeavor, a creative outlet, *and* a necessary survival act.

Have you ever heard the saying, "Eat to live, don't live to eat"? I understand the intention behind the first part of the saying—put food into your body that helps it to thrive—but I have trouble with the second part. Certainly life should be about more than food, and we shouldn't "live to eat," but food is such an integral part of our lives that it demands our attention. We eat multiple times a day and were created to do so. Semantics aside, eating and living go hand-in-hand.

When you really begin eating the way you were meant to eat as outlined in this book, you will notice positive changes in all areas of your life. You will feel better emotionally and physically. You will be empowered by your choices instead of being tossed to and fro by the changing tide of popular diet trends. You will be more in tune with the world and your environment. You may even become involved in the politics of food—choosing to vote with your dollars by joining a community-supported agriculture program (CSA), buying organic food, or even growing a garden of your own.

We were meant to eat and to enjoy it! Enjoyment of food and the pursuit of health need not be mutually exclusive—in fact, that was never the intent. Food is a divine gift that is supposed to be one of the pleasures of life. When it is a source of stress and a cause of poor health, the relationship is broken. My hope for you in reading this book is that you have made steps towards restoring your relationship with food, making it one that allows you to eat the way you were always meant to eat.

ABOUT THE AUTHOR

Lindsay Reinholt is a certified health coach who lives and works in Warsaw, Indiana. As a health coach, she is deeply passionate about helping her clients achieve their unique health goals. She also leads workshops at doctors' offices and corporations. In addition, she serves as a fitness instructor at her local YMCA. There she has developed and teaches exercise programs for moms and babies, allowing new mothers to get back in shape while bonding with their little ones and other moms in a healthy setting.

She received her health coach training through the Institute for Integrative Nutrition and also has degrees in Spanish, Communications & Culture, and Telecommunications from Indiana University. She wears many hats, but her favorites are as wife to her husband Mitch and mom to daughter Winnie and another baby on the way.

Meet Lindsay, learn about her health coaching programs, and sign up to receive her newsletter at www.lindsayreinholt.com.

LINDSAY REINHOLT

SPEAKER HIGHLIGHT

Interested in having Lindsay speak at your next event? Sample topics include:
- Mindful Eating
- Meal Planning
- Feeding Our Families
- The Bitter Side of Sugar
- The Bio-Individuality of Exercise
- Stress Reduction
- Wellness at Work
- Making Healthy Choices at Restaurants
- Goal-Setting and Intentions
- Cooking classes (seasonal menus, specific food items such as ancient grains, green smoothies, vegetarian meals, etc.)

Lindsay is also able to develop custom workshops according to the needs and interests of your organization. Check out her website www.lindsayreinholt.com and contact her at lindsay@lindsayreinholt.com for more information.

LINDSAY REINHOLT

SHARE THE LOVE

Thank you so much for reading this book and allowing me to share in your journey. When I set out to make a career in wellness, I always hoped to have a positive impact on people's lives, but I never imagined having the wide reach that writing a book would give me. The truth is, there are still so many people out there that are struggling. It doesn't take much looking to see a world that is in pain from a broken relationship with food. If you enjoyed this book and felt that its message helped you heal in some way, please consider leaving a review on Amazon. The more reviews, the bigger the reach, and the more people that, like you, can have their lives changed by what they read. Again, thank you, from very the bottom of my heart.

- Lindsay

LINDSAY REINHOLT

NOTES

1. Mann, Traci. *Secrets from the Eating Lab: The Science of Weight Loss, the Myth of Willpower, and Why You Should Never Diet Again.* New York: HarperCollins, 2015. Print.
2. Finkelstein, Lisa M., Rachel L. Frautschy Demuth, and Donna L. Sweeney. "Bias Against Overweight Job Applicants: Further Explorations of When and Why." *Wiley InterScience* 46.2 (2007). Web.
3. Burmeister, Jacob M., Allison E. Kiefner, Robert A. Carels, and Dara R. Musher-Eizenman. "Weight Bias in Graduate School Admissions." *Obesity* 21.5 (2013): 918-920. Web.
4. Arnsten, Amy F. "Stress Signaling Pathways that Impair Prefrontal Cortex Structure and Function." *Nature Reviews Neuroscience* 10.6 (2009): 410-422. Web.
5. Ferdman, Roberto A. "Why Diets Don't Actually Work, According to a Researcher Who Has Studied Them for Decades." *Washington Post.* 4 May 2015. Web.
6. Pietiläinen, K. H., et al. "Does Dieting Make You Fat? A Twin Study." *International Journal of Obesity,* 36 (2012): 454-456. Web.
7. "Junk." Def. 2. *Merriam-Webster.* 2015. Web.
8. Emmons RA, et al. "Counting Blessings Versus Burdens: An Experimental Investigation of Gratitude and Subjective Well-Being in Daily Life," *Journal of Personality and Social Psychology* 84.2 (2003): 377–389. Web
9. "Plant Uses/Edible." *Plants for a Future.* Plants for a Future. 2012. Web.

31122910R00104

Made in the USA
Middletown, DE
20 April 2016